Unusual
Encounters

Unusual Encounters

MEDICINE, SHAKESPEARE, AND HISTORICAL MOMENTS

EDWARD TABOR

North Station Press
Bethesda, Maryland

For more information contact: northstationpress@gmail.com

The following essays originally appeared in these publications:

Economic Botany: "Plant Poisons in Shakespeare"

Harvard Magazine: "When Paintings of Shakespeare's Plants Were Found Behind a Shelf of Books," "A Shakespeare Expert on the Internet, by Surprise," "Harvard Scholars in English"

Hektoen International: "The Night the Emergency Room Staff Vanished," "A Hispanic Amulet Against Disease in Infants," "Learning the Vocabulary of Medicine (and Other Foreign Languages)," "Scientific Discoveries in Dreams: Sleeping While the Mind Works," "Will DNA be the Next Invisible Ink?," "Research Opportunities for Medical Students and Residents," "The Origins of NIH Medical Research Grants," "Medical Misinformation and 'The Bellman's Fallacy' in the Internet Era," "Long Before Pearl Harbor, an Entire Hospital Was Sent to Help England in World War II"

History Cambridge: "The Mystery Plaque"

ISBN: 979-8-9904404-0-1 (Paperback)
ISBN: 979-8-9904404-1-8 (Hardback)

Printed in the U.S.A.

Contents

Medicine and Science

1. The Night the Emergency Room Staff Vanished   3
2. A Hispanic Amulet Against Disease in Infants   7
3. Learning the Vocabulary of Medicine (and Other Foreign Languages)   11
4. Scientific Discoveries in Dreams: Sleeping While the Mind Works   17
5. Will DNA be the Next Invisible Ink?   25
6. Research Opportunities for Medical Students and Residents   29
7. The Origins of NIH Medical Research Grants   33
8. Medical Misinformation and "The Bellman's Fallacy" in the Internet Era   47

Shakespeare

9. When Paintings of Shakespeare's Plants Were Found Behind a Shelf of Books   53
10. A Shakespeare Expert on the Internet, by Surprise   59

11. Plant Poisons in Shakespeare 63

12. The Politician Who Loved Shakespeare 87

13. Mr. Siegel Was King Lear 95

14. Shakespeare's Bilingual Play 99

15. Shakespeare and Memory 105

Historical Moments

16. Justice Souter 113

17. Harvard Scholars in English 117

18. The Mystery Plaque 121

19. Long Before Pearl Harbor, an Entire Hospital Was Sent to Help England in World War II 129

20. A Harvard Class in World War II 137

21. Things I Noticed on the Day Robert Kennedy Was Buried 151

22. The Obituary Reader 155

23. Obituaries of Spies 161

24. African Slaves in the North 167

25. Two Great European Writers Who Were Descendants of African Slaves 173

26. Time and Punishment 181

References, Notes, and Sources

References, Notes, and Sources 187

Medicine and Science

The Night the Emergency Room Staff Vanished

One of the strangest events of my medical career occurred on a spring evening in 1975. It was during one of my outpatient months as a pediatric resident at a large medical center in New York City. During the day, I took care of infants, children, and adolescents in the pediatric clinic; at night, I saw pediatric patients in the main emergency room (ER).

On this particular evening, the ER was fairly quiet. I sent home my last patient around 11 p.m. and there were no more patients for me to examine. I headed toward the on-call room upstairs to try to sleep for an hour or two after I told the head nurse to call me when any more patients came in.

On my way out of the ER, I walked past the open door to a small room in the back known as "the kitchen." Nurses, attendants, and secretaries often brought cookies or a cake from home to leave on the counter for their colleagues to eat. This evening, there were two beautiful lasagna casseroles. I looked at the thick sprinkles of ground parsley on top of the light-yellow pasta. The lasagnas were pristine: neither had been cut into yet.

I was tempted: a resident is always hungry because it is often impossible to eat at normal mealtimes when you are busy. I would always eat whatever food was lying around, but on this evening I wanted to get some sleep, so I resisted the temptation.

At 3 a.m. the phone in my on-call room rang and someone told me that a new patient had arrived for me in the ER. (In 1975 we did not have pagers yet for most of the doctors in the hospital.)

When I re-entered the ER a few minutes later, I immediately noticed an eerie silence. I could not find any doctors or nurses near the nurses' station or in the examining areas. As I continued looking around, I began to feel as if I were in a "last man on earth" movie, but I told myself that there must be a nurse somewhere, since I assumed it had been a nurse who had phoned me. When I finally found a nurse, it was someone I had never seen before.

She told me that the entire night staff in the ER had been overcome by an intoxication. I had left the ER at 11 p.m., and around midnight the head nurse had walked over to another part of the hospital to see the hospital's nursing supervisor, to complain that she could no longer work in the ER because "everyone there is laughing at me."

The supervisor went to investigate and found many of the ER staff laughing uncontrollably. Some also could no longer stand up. She found the ER's radiologist sitting in front of the x-ray viewing screen, mesmerized by an x-ray in which he told her the heart was beating. In the ambulance bay, she found a driver revving the engine but going nowhere.

The nursing supervisor called for assistance and found beds for all of the staff, most of whom soon fell asleep. She arranged for a small number of substitute doctors and nurses from other parts of the hospital. She also found someone to phone all patients who had been sent home earlier that night to make sure that no illnesses were missed, and she arranged for physicians to check the patient records and x-rays. The only error discovered was the misreading of one x-ray, and that patient was called back in.

It did not take her long to realize that there had been marijuana in the lasagna in the ER kitchen, and everyone on the ER staff had eaten some of it. Later in the morning, the city police found out further details.

A nurse on the night shift had been at a party before going to work, and he had brought the two lasagna casseroles. The parsley sprinkles turned out to be marijuana. He told the police that he had come to work directly from the party and had asked his host if he could take some food to share with his coworkers in the ER. The police believed his claim that he had not known about the marijuana, and they said there was no evidence that anyone else had tried to target the hospital.

This occurred at a time when marijuana was illegal in all US states, although it was nevertheless widely available. Today, however, it is even more widely available, because marijuana is now legal for recreational use in 39 states and the District of Columbia.

The work of an entire hospital unit was disrupted for many hours because someone naively brought in food from a questionable outside source, and because almost 100% of the ER staff ate some of it. The lives of many patients were placed at risk that night, although fortunately no one was harmed.

2

A Hispanic Amulet
Against Disease in Infants

In my pediatric residency at a New York City hospital many years ago, I noticed that half of my Hispanic infant patients, as well as some toddlers, wore a small black and red amulet that their parents hoped would protect against disease. When I asked other residents and attending physicians about it, none of them seemed to know anything about it. I became curious about the origin of this amulet, but I was not able to find it out until recently.

As a resident, I began asking the parents of my patients about the amulet while I began each physical examination. It was an excellent conversation opener; the parents seemed to relax when they talked about it. I kept records of many of those conversations.

They told me that the amulet is called an "azabache." They told me it would guard against "the evil eye" ("mal de ojo"), and they named the diseases of childhood that it could prevent: diarrhea, respiratory infections, deformities, and, particularly, sudden infant death. As one mother explained it, "Of course it works. He's never been sick before this."

The word "azabache" is Spanish for "jet," a minor gemstone that is one of the substances used to make the amulet. The amulet was worn either on a gold chain on the wrist or occasionally pinned to the undershirt over the left breast with a small safety pin. It came in two forms: One was a small black fist, about 8 mm in length, often with a small red bead on the proximal end; in most cases, the thumb of the fist was tucked under the forefinger. The second form was a black polyhedron about 3 to 4 mm in diameter, paired with a smaller red bead. Among those who wore it, 29% wore the fist and 71% wore the polyhedron. The parents maintained there was no difference in significance between the two forms.

It was purchased for the baby by the parents, grandparents, or other relatives, but the parents told me that it was always purchased *after* the birth of the baby. At that time, an azabache cost between $3 to $10 in folk medicine stores called "botanicas;" today, an azabache can be bought on the internet for between $9 to $55 (without the chain). In my clinic, 40% of babies with an azabache also wore a Virgin Mary medallion.

I wondered about the source of this tradition. Most of these patients lived in neighborhoods where the culture of Puerto Rico was dominant. The culture of Puerto Rico is derived from several converging cultures: Spanish, West African, and Native American (mostly Taino) peoples. A few of these infants wearing the azabache were in families from Cuba or the Dominican Republic, islands that also had been populated by the Taino people before colonization by Spain. In addition to Taino ancestry and colonization by Spain, all three islands had in common an influx of enslaved people brought by the Spanish from sub-Saharan Africa. The black fist made me think the tradition perhaps could have had West African origins.

However, I recently found a short story by Washington Irving (1783–1859) that suggests the amulet probably originated in the Muslim cultures of North Africa. The Moors of North Africa, consisting of Berbers and Arabs, ruled Spain for almost 800 years, from 711 to 1492 AD. Washington Irving's "Legend of the Two Discreet Statues,"[1] a ghostly tale of hidden treasure buried by the Moors in Spain, tells the origin of a similar amulet:

[A young Spanish girl] Sanchica with some of her playmates sported among the ruins of an old Moorish fort that crowns the mountain, when, in gathering pebbles in the fosse, she found a small hand curiously carved of jet, the fingers closed, and the thumb firmly clasped upon them. ... an old tawny soldier drew near, who had served in Africa, and was as swarthy as a Moor. He examined the hand with a knowing look. "I have seen things of this kind," said he, "among the Moors of Barbary. It is a great virtue to guard against the evil eye and all kinds of spells and enchantments." . . . [Her mother] tied the little hand of jet to a ribbon, and hung it round the neck of her daughter.

For three months in 1829, Irving lived in an apartment inside the Alhambra, a Moorish palace in Granada, Spain, whose governor he had befriended. Here, he had access to the palace's staff and archives. He filled his journals with stories and legends about the Moors,[2] which he published in 1832 in *Tales of the Alhambra*.[3] This story indicates that the tradition of the amulet was brought to Spain from the Muslim peoples of North Africa, and one can assume that from Spain it was brought to the Caribbean colonies.

The world is full of risks, and disease is one of the greatest of these. The azabache was placed on an infant to counteract those risks, and it provided the family a sense of control. Today, the existence of numerous websites selling the azabache shows that these beliefs continue.

3

Learning the Vocabulary of Medicine (and Other Foreign Languages)

Both of my parents were physicians and their discussions were often medical. One weekend when I was about 4 years old, I listened to one such conversation at lunch and interrupted to ask, "When I grow up, will I be able to speak the language you speak?" They paused to assure me that I would. In the end, I, too, went to medical school and learned that language.

Learning the vocabulary of medicine is like learning a foreign language. It has been estimated that a medical student learns more than 9,000 new words during the first year[1] and about 55,000 new words during the entire four years of medical school.[2] However, the way these totals were calculated was not reported. In addition, the number of medical words that are actually needed to become a good doctor has never been determined.

Whatever the actual number of words learned per year by medical students, we do not really know the limits of human memory for anything, let alone for medical terms and definitions. The vast majority of medical terms are derived from Latin, and for many generations teachers and parents have advised pre-medical students to study Latin because it is helpful in learning the vocabulary of medicine. Whether this is true or not, it does reflect the similarity between learning the medical vocabulary and learning a foreign language.

We know from various personal accounts a little about the capacity to learn words in a new language, and this might suggest the limits for memorizing medical words. I know a physician whose advisor at a Chinese university told her to study English by buying an English language newspaper every day, from which she memorized 50 English words per day. Even if this were done only on weekdays, it would have been more than 13,000 words per year.

There are a few published accounts of people who were said to have had a large capacity for memorizing foreign words; it is not possible to confirm them. A teacher from Germany who was working in Boston in the 19th century was said to have "had the habit of learning, before breakfast, one hundred words of some foreign language,"[3] which would have been more than 36,000 words per year if true. A British intelligence officer in the years leading up to World War II, F.W. Winterbotham, recorded that German press officers who had been selected to work with foreign journalists were required to memorize 100 English words per week,[4] equal to 5,200 words per year. In the 1980s, a Soviet spy, Oleg Gordievsky, learned 30 English words per day to facilitate his work as a double agent for the UK,[5] equal to almost 11,000 words per year. These examples, taken together, show that some people have the capacity to learn many thousands of words per year.

Learning the vocabulary of medicine may be somewhat easier than learning an actual foreign language. Medical words are learned within a framework of the structure and function of the body or in relation to a disease. The memorized words are reinforced by the framework, as well as by being encountered over and over again in other classes and on the wards. It is important to try to put the words into sentences, practicing everywhere and upon everybody, to assist with retaining the memory.

Learned medical words are reinforced by the context of medicine in the same way that an actor's memorized lines are reinforced by the context of a play, or a musician's memorization of a score is reinforced by the sound of the music. One 20-year-old concert pianist told an interviewer that "it takes her about two weeks, practicing two to three hours a day, to memorize 100 pages of music."[6] She said that she was able to play 20 piano concertos from memory.

For the vocabulary of medicine, case histories provide context that helps with memorizing. Paul Farmer, the founder of the medical philanthropy Partners in Health, known for his encyclopedic medical memory, ascribed it to using case histories as mnemonics. He used the memory of the patient's face, small quirks, and possessions as a framework for remembering symptoms, pathophysiology, and remedies for thousands of diseases.[7]

Medical students have long used mnemonic phrases to help them memorize finite groups of new words. Generations of medical students have memorized the mnemonic "On Old Olympus's towering tops . . . " to remember the cranial nerves, as well as other mnemonics, mostly passed along through generations of medical students outside of the classroom, although lists of these have been published online[8] and in books in recent years.

There is some evidence that a person can work to increase their memory capacity, but it is not known whether medical students improve their memorization abilities as they progress in their medical studies. Certainly, the required pre-medical college courses have incidentally pre-selected them for the capacity to memorize large numbers of new words. Psychologists have shown that improving memory capacity is possible, and they have been able to train students to learn increasingly long series of numbers;[9] furthermore, participants in timed memory competitions can train themselves to learn increasingly long strings of numbers.[10]

Another example of increasing one's ability to memorize was described by Sanford Greenberg, an inventor and philanthropist who became blind at age 20 and expanded his memory in order to continue his education. In a memoir, he described learning how to visualize mental lecture notes. "I memorized virtually every sentence read to me that year, something of which I did not know I was capable. ... I had to absorb material in a way I never had before. I still remember much of what I learned then. And I discovered that acquiring knowledge at such an insane pace would be a continuous wonder and joy . . . "[11]

Almost 22,000 new students enter US medical schools every year. When they graduate four years later, they will have mastered tens of thousands of new medical words. They will use this medical vocabulary for the rest of their professional lives: to keep records of patient care, to understand medical journals, to participate in continuing medical education, to communicate with colleagues, and to report new medical findings.

4

Scientific Discoveries in Dreams: Sleeping While the Mind Works

Some major scientific discoveries have been revealed in dreams during sleep. Since ancient times, Western culture has included a deep belief in the power of dreams to provide information. The Greek philosopher Heraclitus (c. 500 BC) spoke of how "even in their sleep men are at work."[1] The Roman emperor Marcus Aurelius (121 AD to 180 AD) noted that he learned about "remedies prescribed for me in dreams—especially in cases of blood-spitting and vertigo."[2] There are also some examples from more recent centuries.

August Kekulé (1829–1896), a German chemist, had been trying to figure out how groups of six carbon atoms could combine to make the organic chemicals that are found in all living beings. While doing so in 1865, he fell asleep in front of a fire and dreamed of a self-devouring snake chasing its tail, and when he awoke, he realized that the six carbon atoms must be joined together in a circle, now called the "benzene ring."[3]

For many years, Kekulé's dream has been well-known to students of chemistry, but it became even more widely known due to its use by the psychiatrist Carl Jung,[3,4,5] although Jung described Kekulé's dream being of the snake with its tail in its mouth. Jung used it as an example of symbols located in the "collective unconscious," his concept of a library of subconscious images within the minds of all humans that he believed we inherited from our prehistoric ancestors.

Dmitri Mendeleev (1834–1907), a Russian chemist,[6] wanted to design a table in which all of the 63 then-known chemical elements[7] would be aligned based on their atomic weights. He had only been able to align about thirty elements until one night when he had a dream in which he saw almost all of the 63 elements in a large tabular arrangement, a "periodic table." The next morning, he wrote it down. In 2001, the historian of science Oliver Sacks examined Mendeleev's drafts of the table and asserted that "Mendeleev did not wake from his dream with all the answers in place, but, more interestingly, perhaps, woke with a sense of revelation, so that within hours he was able to solve many of the questions that had occupied him for years."[6]

Louis Agassiz (1807–1873), a prominent biologist at Harvard University, discovered the structure of a certain prehistoric fish by means of a recurring dream. In 1832, when he was 25 years old, he had been trying for two weeks to figure out what kind of fish had made a small fossilized impression on a stone slab. He awoke one night and realized that he had seen the fish in his sleep with all the missing features. He tried to hold onto the image in his mind, but it vanished. During the day, he continued to try to retrieve the image without success. The next night, he dreamed of the fish again, but with the same outcome when he awoke. On the third night, he put a paper and pencil next to his bed. As morning neared, the fish appeared again in a dream. Then, according to a posthumous biography written by his wife,[8] "still half dreaming, in perfect darkness he traced these characters [of the fish] on the sheet of paper at the bedside." In the morning, using the drawing as his guide, "he succeeded in chiseling away the surface of the stone under which portions of the fossilized fish proved to be hidden. When wholly exposed, it corresponded with his dream and his drawing, and he succeeded in classifying it with ease."[8]

Otto Loewi (1873–1961), a German physiologist and pharmacologist, discovered in a dream how to show that chemicals transmit nerve messages across nerve junctions.[9] In 1903, he had had the idea that nerve transmission might occur by means of chemicals, but he could not then think of an experiment to show this. Seventeen years later, on two successive nights in 1920, he dreamed of a laboratory experiment that would allow him to verify his earlier hypothesis.[9] On the first night, he awoke and wrote down the dream. In the morning, he was certain he had dreamed something important, but he could not remember it and could not decipher his writing. On the next night, he awoke at 3 a.m. and realized he had dreamed it again. By his own account, he "got up immediately, went to the laboratory, and performed a simple experiment on a frog heart according to the nocturnal design. ... its results became the foundation of the theory of chemical transmission of the nervous impulse."[9] For this discovery, he shared the Nobel Prize in Physiology or Medicine with Sir Henry Dale in 1936.

Loewi's analysis of this experience provides some insight into how dreams can lead to scientific discoveries:

> The story of this discovery shows that an idea may sleep for decades in the unconscious mind and then suddenly return. Further, it indicates that we should sometimes trust a sudden intuition without too much skepticism. If carefully considered in the daytime, I would undoubtedly have rejected the kind of experiment I performed. ... It was good fortune that at the moment of the hunch I did not think but acted immediately.[9]

To further complicate this experience, 35 years later, around 1955, he came across a paper he had written in 1918 using a similar experiment for a different purpose.

He then concluded that the dream in 1920 represented the subconscious association of the hypothesis of 1903 with the method tested in 1918.

Srinivasa Ramanujan (1887–1920) was an Indian mathematical genius who went from poverty in southern India to work at Cambridge University in the United Kingdom and received the highest honors in world mathematics. He told a friend that the Hindu goddess Namagiri gave him mathematical insights in his dreams. He told another friend that in his dreams he saw drops of blood associated with the god Narasimha, the male consort of Namagiri, after which "scrolls containing the most complicated mathematics used to unfold before his eyes."[10] However, one of his biographers expressed doubts whether he really believed that his ideas came in dreams.[10]

Henri Poincaré (1854–1912), a prominent French mathematician, reported that solutions to mathematical problems often "come to me in the morning or evening in my bed while in a semi-hypnagogic state."[11] Hypnagogic sleep[12] is a drowsy state that sometimes occurs during the transition from waking to sleep and often includes episodic dream-like visions. However, the visions of these states differ from actual dreams in having less emotional content. As in dreams, however, the working of subconscious ideas can be released from the inhibitions of consciousness during hypnagogic states. Poincaré said that these kinds of scientific inspirations came to him throughout his life with some regularity. He described one such occasion when "ideas arose in crowds; I sensed them colliding with each other, until two of them linked up together, as it were, to form a stable combination." The next morning, he found that he had the solution to a problem with which he had been struggling for two weeks.[11]

Discussion

Most scientific solutions do not arrive in dreams. Every year, thousands of important scientific problems are solved by thousands of scientists around the world, mostly as a result of dedicated sustained work and careful thinking. A few may result from sudden inspirations during waking hours, and even fewer from dreams.

Most of the dreams discussed here occurred to people who were thinking deeply about a specific problem during their waking hours. It is possible that such dreams may only occur in the context of intensive scientific thinking.

Nevertheless, solutions to scientific problems in dreams or in a hypnagogic state may occur more often than we realize. It is very difficult to remember any dreams even a few seconds after awaking, and scientific solutions might be found more often in dreams if more people remembered their dreams after awaking.

The subconscious mind is constantly at work, during waking and sleeping, linking different ideas that the dreamer has not seen connections between. The dream, if remembered on awaking, reveals those connections to the conscious mind. Carl Jung likened these dream revelations to the sudden flash of insight from the subconscious mind of a genius. He wrote that "the capacity of the human psyche to produce such new material is particularly significant when one is dealing with dream symbolism, for I have found again and again in my professional work that the images and ideas that dreams contain . . . [sometimes] express new thoughts that have never yet reached the threshold of consciousness."[5]

Dreams, of course, no matter how insightful, are not a substitute for further research and experimental proof. Kekulé insisted it was important to verify the ideas revealed in dreams and that we should "beware of publishing our dreams before they have been examined by the conscious understanding."[11]

5

Will DNA be the Next Invisible Ink?

Deoxyribonucleic acid (DNA), the chemical that forms our genes, can be used to encode and transmit narrative documents and photos, as shown in several published studies. DNA might also become the next "invisible ink" because messages in DNA can be "hidden in plain sight" to reduce the chance of being detected.

Most research on DNA for storing narrative information has focused on meeting society's future needs for archival storage. Scientists at Harvard University coded a genetics book in DNA (including 53,426 words and 11 JPG images),[1] created 70 billion DNA copies of the book, and then translated it back into English. Scientists at the European Bioinformatics Institute (EBI) in the UK coded in DNA all of Shakespeare's sonnets (in ASCII text), a color photo (in JPG format), a scientific paper (in PDF format), and a recording of a speech (in MP3 format). They created 12 million copies and sent the DNA to another laboratory where it was decoded.

All of the files were back to their original condition, and the sonnets could again be read in English.[2] In each of these studies, there were few coding errors,[1,2] in part due to the large number of DNA copies made, which permitted checking for accuracy. DNA is ideal for this: one gram of single-stranded DNA can hold more than 215 petabytes of data,[3] equal to the capacity of 300 million compact discs, but occupies a volume smaller than a poppyseed.[4] A shorter message would be essentially invisible to the naked eye.

How does this work? Genetic information in living cells is coded in DNA by means of four chemicals: adenine, thiamine, guanine, and cytosine (abbreviated by the letters A, T, G, and C), arranged in groups of three. For instance, the triplet "TAC" encodes the amino acid methionine. To code a narrative message, there are 64 possible permutations of A, T, G, and C in groups of three. Twenty-six of these can be selected to code the 26 letters of the English alphabet (or any other alphabet), and the remaining unused permutations can be used to code dummy letters to make the code more difficult to break. Alternatively, the binary system of digital data storage using "0's" and "1's" can be converted to DNA coding. For instance, "A" and "C" can be used interchangeably to mean "0" and "G" and "T" interchangeably to mean "1," as done in the Harvard study.[1] Software to do this, developed by others under the aegis of a US government research program, the Molecular Information Storage program of the Intelligence Advanced Research Projects Activity (IARPA), has also been reported.[4]

The message is coded in the form of overlapping segments of DNA, rather than one large DNA molecule. The Harvard study used 159-nucleotide segments[1] and the EBI study used 117-nucleotide segments.[2] Each segment also includes coded indexing details to show where it fits into the larger message. Overlapping segments provide duplicate copies of the message and thus serve to safeguard the coding accuracy. The DNA for coding these messages can be synthesized without the use of a pre-existing strand of DNA as a template, making the process simpler than natural DNA synthesis in a cell.[3]

Throughout history, invisible inks, and later microdots, were used to hide coded messages. In a similar way, DNA-encoded messages "hidden in plain sight" can prevent, or at least delay, attempts by outsiders to decode them. For instance, DNA messages placed in dried saliva on the gummed seals of envelopes would be undetected unless someone knew that this contained a coded message. A smudge of DNA can be hidden on a scrap of tissue or a piece of clothing, particularly if hidden in the midst of other DNA smudges. Only the intended recipient would know where to look for it and what DNA primers to use to amplify the message.

Hiding the message requires minimal effort. DNA is hardy; it is not destroyed by long storage, cold temperatures, or mild heat, particularly if the fragments are short.

Dry DNA is often readable after thousands of years in the ground.[5] In addition, methods have been developed to make DNA stable even in wet conditions by creating "mirror image DNA"[6] (with "L" chirality instead of the "D" chirality of natural DNA), which cannot be degraded by normal enzymes found in the environment.

Portable equipment is available to decode messages in DNA. A handheld DNA sequencer can be as small as four inches long, weighing 90 grams, and can be plugged into a laptop. Thus, DNA messages can be read almost anywhere, allowing a government agency to send messages to its agents in the field.

The use of DNA for storing non-genetic data has been reported in the scientific literature. Thus, it is likely that the methods described here have already been attempted for sending messages in secrecy. Countermeasures will no doubt be sought, such as ways to differentiate artificial DNA from natural DNA in everyday locations. This might be difficult because of the ubiquity of natural DNA in our environment, and intercepting specific messages might have to rely on information from double agents or from intercepted communications regarding the locations of DNA-encoded messages.

6

Research Opportunities
for Medical Students and Residents

Medical students and residents who engage in scientific research obtain numerous advantages that may enhance their careers. They acquire analytical skills, refine their critical thinking, and may obtain better future training opportunities. Unfortunately, scientific research is often not part of their training, leading to the suggestion that this should change and that some scientific research opportunities should be included in current medical residency programs.[1]

There is also the additional potential benefit that by participating in research, students or residents may make important advances in medicine, as shown by a few advances described here.

Cardiac catheterization: Werner Forssmann (1904–1979) was a surgical intern in Eberswalde, Germany, a small town fifty miles from Berlin, when in 1929 he had

the idea of introducing a catheter into the heart by way
of an antecubital vein, which eventually led to the development of cardiac catheterization. His department chairman refused to give him permission to try this either on
patients or on himself. As recounted by Steckelberg et al.,
he tried it anyway, first on cadavers and then on himself:

> . . . after deceiving the surgical nurse into thinking
> that she would be the subject, and thus gaining access
> to the necessary sterile instruments, he persuaded her
> into allowing herself to be tied to the operating table
> (preventing her from interfering with his plans), anes-
> thetized his own left cubital fossa, advanced the cath-
> eter into his right atrium, and then climbed several
> flights of stairs to the x-ray department to document
> his achievement.[2]

One of his fellow residents later recalled, "I remember so
well the day when Werner Forssmann came a little later
than usual to our luncheon round table . . . Forssmann
told us that he was a little bit delayed because he had just
put a ureteral [*sic*] catheter from his left arm into the right
ventricle . . . "[3] The x-ray of the catheter in his own right
atrium was published with a description of the work in
Klinische Wochenshrift. However, his findings were not
accepted by the medical community; he conducted further
studies for two more years but spent the years after 1931 as
a surgeon in various undistinguished posts and as a "country doctor." When he won the Nobel Prize for the catheter
work twenty-seven years later (in 1956, with Cournand and

Richards), the presentation speech said Forssmann's work was proof "that – even in our enlightened times – a valuable suggestion may remain unexploited on the grounds of a preconceived opinion."[2]

Antibiotics for treating ulcers: Barry Marshall (1951–) was a resident in internal medicine in Australia when a supervisor called his attention to twenty patients whose stomach biopsies contained curved bacteria. Marshall and others worked for eight months to culture the bacteria, and within a year had found that these bacteria were present in all patients with duodenal ulcers and in 80% of patients with gastric ulcers. The bacterium was *Helicobacter pylori,* and this discovery led to the ability to treat gastric ulcers with antibiotics. Marshall experimentally induced gastritis in himself by ingesting the bacteria, and cured it with antibiotics. He subsequently confirmed the findings in controlled clinical trials of antibiotics in conjunction with antacids to treat patients with duodenal ulcers.[4] He was awarded the Nobel Prize for the work in 2005.

Bromsulphthalein (BSP) clearance test for liver function: Sanford M. Rosenthal (1897–1989) invented the bromsulphthalein (BSP) clearance test for evaluating liver function, based on an idea he had while a medical student at Vanderbilt University. He had read about earlier studies of liver clearance of a dye in which the dye had to be measured in the stool, which was too cumbersome and messy to be clinically useful.[5] He had the then-novel idea that it might be possible to determine clearance by measuring how much of a dye remained in the blood, and thus determine if liver function were impaired. However, he was not able to develop the practical use of the idea until after he completed his internship.[5,6,7] The BSP became the primary test for clinical liver function, and remained so until the development of enzyme tests for liver function in the 1960s.

Discovery of insulin: Charles Best (1899–1978)[8] was a medical student at the University of Toronto when he and Frederick Banting discovered insulin. For Best, the work began as a summer project just before starting medical school in 1921, assisting Banting in the laboratory of J.J.R. Macleod. He continued to work intensively on the project while a medical student during the following year; the work was publicly presented in December 1921 and published in February 1922 under the names of Banting and Best. Although the Nobel Prize was awarded to Banting and Macleod in 1923, the medical community and history have always correctly referred to the discovery of insulin "by Banting and Best."

These examples of major medical breakthroughs brought about by scientific thinking and research conducted by medical students and residents provide support for including at least some research opportunities as part of medical school and residency programs.

7

The Origins of NIH
Medical Research Grants

The US National Institutes of Health (NIH) supports medical research in non-government universities and hospitals, and some small businesses. The cost and scope of these grants significantly exceed those of NIH's own intramural program of clinics, wards, and laboratories. The NIH extramural grants today provide more than \$37 billion[1,2] for 50,000[2] new and ongoing grants each year. These grants have led to many of the most important discoveries in medicine and the biological sciences in the past century. This grants program developed from the US government's efforts to marshal science resources for World War II. Thus, preparations for war incidentally brought about great benefits in health.

The Beginnings: Medical Research Contracts for World War II

The US government generally did not pay for medical research outside of its own laboratories before 1938, with rare exceptions.[3,4] Most medical research in the US had been supported by pharmaceutical companies and a few private foundations, most notably the Rockefeller Foundation. By 1934, the Rockefeller Foundation provided two-thirds of all funding for medical and public health research in the US.[5] In 1930, Congress created the "National Institute of Health" (later renamed the "National Institutes of Health;" the abbreviation "NIH" will be used here for both) by renaming the "Hygienic Laboratory" of the US Public Health Service (USPHS). It was conceived on a relatively small scale, but a series of additional laws passed by Congress during the 1930s and 1940s enlarged the structure of NIH, which ultimately affected the nature of the future grants program. (Table 1)

As World War II began in Europe, James Conant, president of Harvard University, had the idea of creating a government committee to stimulate scientific research for military preparedness. He brought the idea to Vannevar Bush, head of the Carnegie Institution, and Bush brought the idea to President Franklin Roosevelt. In 1940, Roosevelt created the National Defense Research Committee (NDRC), with Vannevar Bush as its head, to oversee war-related scientific research and to award research contracts to civilian universities and institutes.

Table 1. Laws and Events that Shaped the NIH Grants Program

Year	Law	Action
1930	Ransdell Act	Created NIH within USPHS
1937	National Cancer Act	Created NCI within USPHS but independent of NIH
1938–1940		NIH and NCI moved to Bethesda campus
1944	Public Health Service Act of 1944 (PL410)	Moved NCI into NIH; authorized USPHS (NIH) grants to universities and hospitals[a]
1948	National Heart Act	Created heart and dental institutes at NIH; renamed NIH as "National Institutes of Health"

Abbreviations in Table 1: NCI = National Cancer Institute; NIH = National Institute(s) of Health; USPHS = US Public Health Service

[a] Separately, a small number of cancer research grants had been issued by NCI since 1938, as authorized by the National Cancer Act of 1937.

In June 1941, at Bush's suggestion, Roosevelt created the Office of Scientific Research and Development

(OSRD) to oversee NDRC, with Bush as head. Conant now became head of NDRC, a position in which he later coordinated the US development of the atomic bomb. At the same time, a Committee on Medical Research (CMR) was created under OSRD to review medical needs and proposed medical research contracts. The director of CMR was Alfred N. Richards, who had been Vice President of Medical Affairs at the University of Pennsylvania and a noted pharmacologist and researcher on kidney disease. CMR members included Dr. Rolla Eugene Dyer, director of NIH (representing the Surgeon General of the USPHS), as well as the Surgeons General of the Army and Navy, and others.

But CMR did not give grants for medical research, only contracts.[6] CMR was concerned mainly with solutions to specific problems, and contracts gave the government more control of the projects, with the goals more clearly spelled out than would be the case for grants.[6] However, these contracts differed from conventional military procurement contracts, because the end products were studies, of which the outcomes were unknown.

Supporting Medical Research in Peacetime

Many people wanted government support of medical research to continue after the war. There was also a growing belief that good medical research could best be obtained by grants to researchers in universities and hospitals rather than contracts, based in part on the success of a small National Cancer Institute (NCI) grants program for cancer research that began in 1938, before NCI was part of NIH (Table 1). In July 1944, with the end of the war in sight, President Roosevelt signed the Public Health Service Act of 1944, which authorized the USPHS to "make grants in aid to universities, hospitals, laboratories, and other public or private institutions, and to individuals."[7]

Also in 1944, Bush wanted to end the CMR program for medical research contracts, and Dyer suggested that these contracts become part of the NIH portfolio.[5,6] NIH converted the contracts to grants at the end of 1945,[8] which helped establish the principle of using grants for medical research. By the end of 1946, the extramural grants run by NCI also became part of the overall NIH research grants portfolio.[8] CMR was disbanded on December 31, 1946.[9]

In 1945, NIH created the Office of Research Grants (changed in 1946 to the Division of Research Grants). Dr. Cassius J. Van Slyke was appointed director on January 1, 1946. Van Slyke had recently come to NIH to work on venereal disease research, but had a heart attack in 1945. Dyer thought that directing the new grants program might be suitable for Van Slyke during his recovery. Van Slyke later quipped that Dyer thought it would be "an incidental part time, left hand, lower drawer of the desk sort of activity."[5] It soon became apparent that it would be a major undertaking and Van Slyke was spending 12 to 14 hours a day on it.[8] Van Slyke remained head of the Division of Research Grants until 1948.

Van Slyke predicted that the NIH grants "may have early and profound effects upon the course of medical history and the national health" and would result in "enormous savings of public and private money" by preventing and curing diseases.[10] Working with a small staff, Van Slyke created the administrative structure and the grants procedures that would remain in use for the next three-quarters of a century. In the beginning, the Office of Research Grants consisted of Van Slyke, his assistant Ernest Allen, and two secretaries. The first grant applications under the new system were solicited by a letter from Van Slyke and Allen to the deans of all US medical schools.

The first new NIH grant[5] was awarded in 1945 (for fiscal year [FY] 1946) for a study at the University of Utah of the inheritance of muscular dystrophy. Money to support this study had been attached to the budget by a Senator from Utah, for $92,000 ($1.5 million in 2022 dollars[11]). Dyer deliberately selected this study for the first use of the new grant-giving authority, and he had it reviewed by the National Advisory Health Council (NAHC), the main NIH advisory council at that time. (A second proposal considered at the same meeting of the NAHC was rejected.)

Initially, the grant funds were only given for one year at a time; research projects lasting longer than one year required submission of a new application each year. These subsequent applications were subject to the same review process, but with the understanding that they would be reviewed favorably as long as progress was being made. Investigators were free to change the research plan and to change the planned expenditures without restriction, as long as the funds were used for research and in accordance with their university's rules. Equipment purchased with grant funds remained the property of the grantee institution after the end of the grant.[10,12]

Expansion of NIH Grants

By the end of 1946, the main processes of the NIH extramural grant program were in place, and were very close in design to those still used today. Almost immediately after the creation of the grants program, it began to expand (Table 2, 3). By October 1946, NIH had funded 264 extramural research grants for a total of $3,900,000 ($55 million in 2022 dollars) at 77 universities in 26 states (including the projects transferred from CMR).[10] By 1951, 25% of medical research publications originating in colleges and universities included acknowledgement of at least some USPHS (i.e. NIH) support; however, at the time, individual NIH grants often provided only partial support.[18] By 1955, NIH was awarding $54 million per year in grants for research, training, and construction of research facilities[8] ($599 million in 2022 dollars). In the words of one writer, "By 1950, the team was in place, the premises were established, the purposes rolled easily off all administrators' tongues; the system was ready and rolling."[8]

Table 2. Growth of Study Sections

Year	Number of Study Sections	Number of Reviewers
1946[8,10]	21	>250
1974[13]	38	677[4]
1987[8]	67	2,200
2022[14]	>250	>18,000

Most NIH research grants were "Research Project Grants," later called "R01 grants." Each supported an individual lead investigator's research project. Other types of grants, including training grants, program project grants, and small business grants, were added later. However, R01 grants always represented a majority of the grants.[1,16]

The expansion of extramural grant funding and the expansion of the number of NIH institutes (each institute dedicated to a specific disease area) occurred in parallel. By 1950, NIH had 6 institutes. The number of institutes continued to increase, reaching 15 by 1970 and 27 by 1998. Each institute had a role in seeking and funding grants in its disease area.

Creating a System to Review Grant Applications

There was a philosophy at NIH that all grant applications should be reviewed by experts from outside the government to avoid potential restriction of scientific innovation and conflicts of interest. This concept of outside review of grants may have been inspired by a temporary federal program in 1879–1883, when a National Health Board gave federal grants to universities for yellow fever research, under the oversight of a committee with a majority of nongovernmental members.[4] More directly, the concept was influenced by the success of the peer-review system that had been set-up by CMR for its medical research contracts.[4] In addition, the Public Health Service Act of 1944 had specified that outside experts should review USPHS (NIH) grants.

To find expert reviewers for the first grant applications, Van Slyke and Allen used a copy of the directory *American Men of Science* to identify potential reviewers among experts in each subject area. In the beginning, Allen recalled, "we would write to three or four of these people and get their opinions on the merit of the proposal. We then took [their assessments of] the proposals to the National Advisory Health Council."[8]

NIH quickly developed a formal two-tiered system of review. Grant applications were submitted to the Division of Research Grants. Then the first level of review was conducted by "study sections" of outside experts, who met in person to review, suggest changes, and (in the early years) to approve or disapprove the applications. By 1950, an early version of a rating system was implemented, whereby study sections gave each application a numerical score instead of recommending approval or disapproval, which permitted funding to be given in order of appraised merit.[4] The number of study sections steadily increased to address the increasing numbers of applications (Table 2). In addition, the study sections were expected to survey the existing research in their subjects in order to find neglected areas in which to encourage future research. Most of the study sections met quarterly, a few weeks in advance of the quarterly meetings of the relevant advisory council. Each study section was coordinated by an "executive secretary;" initially these included some NIH intramural laboratory scientists, but soon these were replaced by fulltime executive secretaries.

Initially, a second-level review was performed by outside experts on one of the three NIH advisory councils: the National Advisory Cancer Council, the National Advisory Mental Health Council, or NAHC for all other research areas.[10] By 1955, each of the eight NIH institutes in existence at that time had its own advisory council of outside experts to conduct the second level of review for grants in their disease areas.[8] The study sections and the advisory councils also formulated research policy by means of the criteria they used to select which grant applications to approve and fund.

NIH Research Grants Today

Today, NIH grants make up more than 84% of the $45 billion FY 2022 NIH budget, or more than $37 billion.[2] (Table 3) These funds support 50,000 new and ongoing grants and more than 300,000 scientists.[2]

Table 3. Growth of Expenditures for NIH Extramural Grants: A Historical Overview

Fiscal Year[a]	Total Cost of NIH Grants	Total in 2022 Dollars[11]
1946[10]	$ 3.9 million	$ 63 million
1956[8]	$ 54 million	$ 599 million
1974[4]	$ 604 million	$ 3.8 billion
1987[4]	$ 2.4 billion	$ 6.4 billion
2022[2]	$ 37 billion	$ 37 billion

[a] The US government's fiscal year ran from July 1 to June 30 in the years from 1842 through 1976, and from October 1 through September 30 from 1977 to the present.[15]

NIH grants are now overseen by the Center for Scientific Review, which interfaces with the 24 NIH institutes and centers that give grants (of a total of 27 institutes and centers). Study sections are now officially called "scientific review groups" although the term "study section" is still widely used. The executive secretaries are now called "scientific review officers." Today, study section meetings typically are held about three months before the relevant advisory council meeting;[17] applications are reviewed and given a numerical ranking. The applications are then sent to that institute's advisory council for a secondary review.

Most applications today are investigator-initiated, in which the applicant conceived and developed the research idea. Other applications are submitted in response to an announcement by the relevant NIH institute or center seeking applications for research on a specific medical problem. An "R01" grant application supporting an individual investigator's project[16] can be either investigator-initiated or submitted in response to an announcement, and the grant has a three- to five-year duration.

Conclusions

The NIH medical research grants program arose from a World War II program for medical research contracts. The grants were designed to encourage independent research on important medical and biological topics, and in this they have exceeded expectations. They have funded many of the most important medical advances of our times.

These successes have been due, in part, to the guiding philosophy of the program. As stated by Van Slyke, the NIH grants should be "a medical research program of scientists and by scientists" that maintains "the integrity and independence of the research worker and his freedom from control, direction, regimentation, and outside interference."[10]

8

Medical Misinformation and "The Bellman's Fallacy" in the Internet Era

"The Bellman's Fallacy" is a form of biased thinking in which something is believed to be true because it has been repeatedly stated. Its name comes from the Bellman in Lewis Carroll's "The Hunting of the Snark," who says, "What I tell you three times is true."[1] Based on this poem, the phrase itself was used for many years in non-medical contexts to refer to this type of thinking. (President Theodore Roosevelt occasionally quoted it.[2]) It was given the name "The Bellman's Fallacy" when it was first applied to medical information in 1973.[3,4] Today, the proliferation of medical articles on the internet increases the possibility that this type of faulty thinking will occur.

The term was first used in the medical literature to refer to the incorrect claim that Hippocrates first described lead poisoning, which was reported by several authors who were quoting each other.[4] Later the term was applied to an incorrect statement that undertreatment was the cause of an epidemic of asthma deaths, based on its having been discussed in three earlier publications.[5]

The internet has facilitated the wider occurrence of this potential bias. Many medical headlines and unusual articles result in spin-off articles in countless online publications intended either for medical readers or patients. They turn up in a Google search and sometimes are accepted as true on the basis of multiple citations.

An example of the internet effect occurred in 2023 in a review article by Sahni and Carrus.[6] The authors stated that the growth of "the collective body of medical knowledge required to treat a patient" had a doubling time in 2010 of less than seventy-five days and "today, what medical students learn in their first 3 years would be only 6 per cent of known medical information at the time of their graduation." The doubling time was referenced to an article by Densen,[7] who stated a doubling time of seventy-three days (for 2020, not 2010) and also mentioned the 6% figure, but provided no evidence for either.

A Google search for "doubling time of medical information"[8] found twenty relevant citations, nineteen of which cited Densen's 73-day figure; of these, fourteen referenced the Densen paper and five cited "73 days" without attribution. Thus, the one article by Densen,[7] stating numbers with no evidence basis, was responsible for nineteen Google citations and a further restatement in the Sahni and Carrus review in a prominent journal, making it even more likely to continue being repeated.

It is a normal part of human cognition to accept statements as true when they have been heard repeatedly, but an alert reader must try to avoid doing so without first verifying that the statements are based on data. Familiarity due to having seen something stated multiple times is not easily distinguished from truth because of the "cognitive ease" it provides.[9] Avoiding "The Bellman's Fallacy" has become more difficult in the internet age, but avoiding it should be a goal of every physician reading the medical literature.

Shakespeare

9

When Paintings of Shakespeare's Plants Were Found Behind a Shelf of Books

When Richard Evans Schultes (Harvard A.B. '37, Ph.D. '41) became director of the Botanical Museum of Harvard University in 1967, he could not have imagined that he would soon discover a collection of beautiful paintings hidden behind a shelf of books in the departmental library. These paintings illustrated all of the plants mentioned by Shakespeare, and they showed how extensive Shakespeare's knowledge of botany was.

In the spring semester of 1968, I was a Harvard undergraduate English major looking for a biology course; during the "course shopping period," I sampled and decided to take Schultes' course, "Plants and Human Affairs." Schultes was an "ethnobotanist," someone who studied how different cultures use plants. In fact, he was known as "The Father of Ethnobotany." He was a fascinating teacher, and his course had its own dedicated classroom in the Botanical Museum, a room filled with artifacts he had collected in the Amazon jungles while searching for undiscovered plants. Each year he gave his class a demonstration of how to shoot an Amazonian blowgun that he kept in the classroom.

Schultes had traveled in the jungles of the northwest Amazon region and lived with its indigenous peoples for 12 years before he joined the Harvard faculty. He was collecting plants that were known only to the local tribes and was trying to save that knowledge before it vanished as the tribes adapted to modern cultures. He was particularly interested in plants with possible medicinal uses, such as arrow poisons that could be used as muscle relaxants for surgery. He described coming out of the jungle at the beginning of World War II to find a request from the U.S. government that he go back into the forest to search for rubber trees, since natural rubber was needed for military airplane tires and the war had cut access to rubber plantations in the South Pacific.

The course required a term paper, and I decided to combine it with my interest in Shakespeare by writing about plant-derived poisons mentioned in Shakespeare's plays. It has always been an axiom at Harvard that if a student can justify an unusual idea, it will be approved, and Schultes welcomed the topic. After I completed the paper, he invited me to submit it for publication in the botanical journal he edited, *Economic Botany*. Thus, I had the opportunity to work with him for the next two years as I revised and polished it for publication.[1] But there was also another reason why Schultes approved my topic.

He confided that he had recently found a spectacular collection of nineteenth-century paintings of Shakespeare's plants hidden behind a row of books in the departmental library. He said that one of his predecessors, Oakes Ames (director of the Botanical Museum from 1923 to 1945) had found the paintings in a bookstall along the Seine during a trip to Paris, had bought the collection, had donated it to the Museum, and then had apparently hidden and forgotten it behind the row of books.

A woman named Rosa M. Towne (1827–1909) had painted these between 1888 and 1898, including all plants Shakespeare mentions in his plays and long poems. In an introductory note to the collection, she wrote that she had decided to do the paintings using "live plants and trees" as models whenever possible. She accompanied each painting by a Shakespeare quotation in which it is mentioned.

The collection comprised 73 paintings of 182 plants, botanically accurate and mostly depicted either in flower or with berries or other fruits. When Shakespeare described several plants in one sentence, she painted these two or three plants in a single painting, artfully assembled but separate enough to appreciate the beauty of each. She also sometimes grouped plants from different plays, such as holly and mistletoe, in this case perhaps because they are both evergreen and associated with Christmas.

Schultes was so impressed by the collection that he decided to look for a publisher to make high-quality reproductions that could be bound as a book. Over the next few years, Schultes updated me about his search for a suitable publisher, a search that took much longer than expected. He often met with publishers while travelling for business or pleasure, including trips to the United Kingdom where he had been most hopeful of finding a suitable publisher, but he could not find one who could meet the high standards of quality that he felt these paintings deserved.

Finally, he found an engraving company in Louisville, Kentucky, which in a test run was able to produce fine reproductions on thick, art-quality paper. Even after the publisher had been selected, production was painstaking and took several years. In 1974, a limited printing of 2,500 copies was published as *Plant Lore of Shakespeare*.[2] Several hundred copies were provided to the Botanical Museum to sell in its gift shop, along with individual unbound pages to be sold as artwork. The proceeds from these sales formed a fund to buy books for the museum's library.

Schultes invited me to the publication party for the book in 1974 at the Pennsylvania Academy of the Fine Arts, where Rosa Towne had once enrolled as an adult student. At the publication party I saw the published book for the first time. It was a large leather-bound folio edition, 15 inches long, a format that is unusual in modern times, even for art books. But a folio was particularly appropriate for a publication related to Shakespeare, since the so-called "First Folio" of his plays contained many works for which no other copies survived. Thus, just as Shakespeare's folio preserved his plays, the folio of Towne's paintings rescued those paintings from obscurity, ensuring their availability for future generations.

The discovery of the Rosa Towne paintings by Oakes Ames, and their rediscovery and publication in book form by Schultes, were important cultural rescues for the future of Shakespeare studies. The book shows the extent of Shakespeare's botanical knowledge, provides a compendium of the 182 plants that we know Shakespeare was familiar with, and lists their common and scientific names. It provided, for the first time, a single collection of botanically accurate paintings that would help scholars and critics visualize exactly what Shakespeare had in mind when he mentioned a plant or when a plant played a key role in the action of one of his plays, such as the plant-derived poison used by Hamlet's uncle to kill Hamlet's father, the king.

I would have loved to own a copy of *Plant Lore of Shakespeare*, but at that time it was selling for $1,000 ($5,200 in 2021 dollars), and that was far beyond what I could afford. Several years later, I must have expressed this wish to Schultes, and he offered to make a copy available to me if I made a cash donation to the Museum. I asked him to inscribe the book before he shipped it to me. His inscription, dated September 16, 1981, read, "Shakespeare means many things to many people. The lover of plants finds him in many ways a worshipper of nature."

10

A Shakespeare Expert
on the Internet, by Surprise

The internet can take you by surprise. I was surprised recently when I discovered that copies of the term paper I wrote for a botany course at Harvard University in 1968 are now being sold online for $39.95 per copy by a major publisher, Springer. In 1970, this term paper, titled "Plant Poisons in Shakespeare," had been published in a botany journal,[1] with the notation, "This article was a term paper in Biology 104 (Plants and Human Affairs) at Harvard College in 1968." Now, 45 years later, someone at Springer decided there is a market for it, but without informing me.

After I found out about this, I ran a Google search and discovered, also to my surprise, that today I am being cited by many Shakespeare websites as an authority on plants in Shakespeare's plays, on the basis of this paper, even though my career has been in a completely different field. "Plant Poisons in Shakespeare" is even listed as extra reading in a Wikipedia article.

To write "Plant Poisons in Shakespeare," I read all 37 of Shakespeare's plays, for the second time during my undergraduate years. (At that time, there were 37 plays known to have been written by William Shakespeare. At the present time, it is generally accepted that he wrote 38 plays.) I made note of the plant poisons that Shakespeare mentioned, and I searched original Elizabethan herbals in Harvard's rare book collection at Houghton Library to document what was believed about these poisons in Shakespeare's time.

Using Houghton Library was a special experience: The library building, with its literary exhibits, was open to the university community, but its reading room was always locked, and readers had to be "buzzed in," which was unusual for any Harvard facility at that time. The room always seemed busy, though hushed; on some days it could be hard to find an empty seat. Most of the readers appeared to be either graduate students or faculty. Special care was enforced to protect the ancient books there. Only pencils were permitted for taking notes; if a reader took a ballpoint pen out of a pocket, a library employee at an elevated desk in the front of the room called out a warning. If a reader's forearm rested on the corner of the book, a similar warning was called out. I quickly learned the process.

Biology 104 was taught by Professor Richard Evans Schultes, who had spent a dozen years searching

Amazonian forests for plants, including those that the Spanish conquistadores had described but that had since disappeared. By 1968 he was not only teaching Biology 104, he was also director of the Harvard Botanical Museum (which since then has been fully absorbed by the Harvard University Museum), and was editor of the journal *Economic Botany*.

Professor Schultes asked me to submit the completed paper to *Economic Botany*, and he asked me to select a few drawings from the original Elizabethan herbals to illustrate my findings. However, Houghton Library would not allow their 1597 edition of Gerarde's *The Herball or Generall Historie of Plantes* to leave the building, even to go to the Fogg Museum where the drawings could be photographed for publication. So Professor Schultes suggested we use a 1636 edition of the same book that he had in the Botanical Museum library. I thus found myself walking down Oxford Street carrying a large book printed in the year that Harvard College was founded, and I was acutely focused on holding it securely and walking carefully.

"Plant Poisons in Shakespeare" also played an unexpected role in another academic event in my life. In the fall of 1968, the person interviewing me for admission to medical school at Columbia University turned out to be the chairman of Columbia's Department of Pharmacology. The interview became a lively discussion of Elizabethan pharmacology, and I have always believed that "Plant Poisons in Shakespeare" played a role in my medical school admission. For many years, I believed that being interviewed by the chairman of Pharmacology was an example of the role of luck in human experience; many years later, however, it occurred to me that he might have been assigned by the admissions committee to interview me, if my application had mentioned the paper, which was in press at the time.

When I learned about Springer selling my paper without my knowledge, I didn't know whether Springer was doing something that was technically legal or not. In the end, I decided not to challenge it for the small amount of monetary compensation I might have been able to get.

Nevertheless, encountering their website selling copies of the paper, and finding Shakespeare websites quoting me about Shakespeare's plants, have been fascinating and unexpected outcomes of a Harvard biology course 45 years ago. It certainly brought back memories of Professor Schultes' office in the Harvard Museum, of my days working in the reading room of Houghton Library with books published before 1600, and of learning how to write a scientific paper in a Harvard course.

11

Plant Poisons in Shakespeare

Plant poisons are pivotal in the action of William Shakespeare's theater. They precipitate plots, as in *Hamlet*; and they culminate plots, as in *Romeo and Juliet*. They indicate Shakespeare's knowledge of plant lore, and they are representative of botanical concepts of the sixteenth and early seventeenth centuries.

Shakespeare's botanical sophistication is at a level near that of the herbalists of the time. Of the duality of plant properties, he writes,

> *Friar Laurence.* Many for many virtues excellent,
> None but for some, and yet all different.
> Oh, mickle is the powerful grace that lies
> In herbs, plants, stones, and their true qualities.
> For naught so vile that on the earth doth live,
> But to the earth some special good doth give;
> Nor aught so good but, strained from that fair use,
> Revolts from true birth, stumbling on abuse.
> Virtue itself turns vice, being misapplied,

And vice sometime's by action dignified.
Within the infant rind of this small flower
Poison hath residence, and medicine power.
For this, being smelt, with that part cheers each part,
Being tasted, slays all senses with the heart.

(*Romeo and Juliet*, II.iii.13–26)[1]

The Elizabethan herbalist Gerarde made a similar observation concerning Crowfoote, *Ranunculus* spp.

For these dangerous simples are likewise many times of themselves beneficiall, and oftentimes profitable: for some of them are not so dangerous, but that they may in some sort, and oftentimes in fit and due season profit and do good.[2(page803)]

Shakespeare may indeed have read some of the herbals that were available before he wrote most of his plays. Banckes' *Herbal*[3] went through 20 known editions between 1525 and 1560. It was popular in London because, unillustrated and printed in quarto and octavo, it was cheaper than its illustrated folio competitors.[4,5] The Turner *Herbal* was published in its first complete edition in 1568.[6] Langham published *The Garden of Health* in 1597.[7] The Frampton translation of Monardes' *Joyfull Newes Out of the New-Found Worlde* appeared in London in 1596.[8] Gerarde's *The Herball or Generall Historie of Plantes* appeared in 1597, incorporating some lore from such earlier herbalists as Turner.[2(page282 et al.)]

Shakespeare may even have been personally acquainted with Gerarde; he may even have seen the herbalist's garden. From 1598 to 1604, while Shakespeare lodged at the corner of Mugwell Street (now Monkswell Street) and Silver Street in Cripplegate,[9,10] Gerarde lived nearby. In 1598, furthermore, Gerarde was examiner of candidates for admission to the Barber-Surgeons' Company in Barber-Surgeons' Hall, almost opposite the corner of Mugwell and Silver Streets.[11] Gerarde describes the type of garden that he and other London herbalists kept.

> These bastard kinds of Flower de-luces, are strangers in England, except it be among some fewe diligent Herbarists in London, who have them in their gardens where they increase exceedingly.[2(page95)]

In addition, one critic points out that for Shakespeare,

> The London to which he went was only a small town by our standards: he could leave it easily on foot and would be rapidly out of it on horse. ... Gerard [*sic*] the Herbalist found many simples 'on the banks of Piccadilla [today's Piccadilly].' ... London was a little urban island amid marsh and forest.[12]

Yet Shakespeare's botanical concepts maintain the spirit of the English countryside; he knew folk plant lore from his childhood in Warwickshire. Throughout his life, he returned to Warwickshire, where he owned property and where, it is thought, his wife remained while he was in London. "He was wont to goe to his native Country once a yeare," the son of one of Shakespeare's fellow actors told the seventeenth century gossip John Aubrey.[13] As an actor, Shakespeare probably toured the countryside during London's plagues; there he would have seen plants and their uses. Also, the night before the Essex insurrection in 1601, Shakespeare's company played *Richard II* with its deposition scene at the request of the Essex faction. When the revolt failed and Shakespeare's former patron Southampton was sent to the Tower, the company at the Globe Theater discreetly went on tour.[14]

Interestingly, the only antidote that is mentioned as such in the plays is Oberon's drug, which removes the effect of Love-in-idleness (the pansy).

> *Oberon.* Then crush this herb into Lysander's eye,
> Whose liquor hath this virtuous property,
> To take from thence all error with his might,
> And make his eyeballs roll with wonted sight.
>
> (*Midsummer Night's Dream*, III.ii.366–369)

Yet the sixteenth century herbals describe dozens of antidotes.[15]

Lust-inducing Drugs

Brabantio. ... thou hast practiced on her with
   foul charms,
Abused her delicate youth with drugs or minerals
That weaken motion.

   (*Othello*, I.ii.73–75; see also *Othello* I.iii.60–61)

The following herbal quotations illustrate some typical
Elizabethan beliefs about lust-inducing drugs.

> [*Solanum melongena*] Madde Apples . . . The people
> of Tolledo do eate them with great devotion being
> boiled with fat flesh, putting thereto some scraped
> cheese, which they do keepe in vineger, honie, or salt
> pickell, all winter to procure lust.[2(page274)]

> [*Iris*, spp.] The Spanish Nut is eaten at the tables of rich
> and delicious, naie vicious persons in sallads, or other-
> wise to procure lust and lecherie.[2(page95)]

> [*Euphorbia*, spp.] Euphorbium . . . Lust to cause,
> stampe it with bayes & arom wel with oile, & anoint
> the virge therwith.[7(page226)]

> [*Urtica*, spp.; *Lamium*, spp.] Nettles . . . The seeds
> drunke with Malmesie provoketh lust, and openeth
> the Matrix. ... Eaten with Onyons and yolkes of egs, it
> moveth Venus.[7(page426)]

> [*Sium sisarum*] The rootes of the Skirret . . . They
> are something windie, by reason whereof they

also provoke lust. ... The women in Swevia, saith *Hieronymus Heroldus*, prepare the roots hereof for their husbands, and knowe full well wherefore and why, &c.[2(page872)]

Certain candied plants were commonly considered lust-inducing, especially the sweet potato, *Ipomoea batatas*. When Shakespeare mentions "potatoes" in the context of inducing lust, scholars believe he is referring to "sweet potatoes."

> *Falstaff.* ... Let the sky rain potatoes. ... hail kissing comfits, and snow eringoes.
>
> (*Merry Wives of Windsor*, V.v.20–22)

> *Thersites.* How the devil luxury, with his fat rump and potato finger, tickles these together!
>
> (*Troilus and Cressida*, V.ii.55–56)

Skirrets (*Sium sisarum*), another root vegetable, was also thought to induce lust. Gerarde says it is

> called of some *Sisarum Peruvianum*, or Skyrrits of Peru . . . or Potatoes . . . notwithstanding howsoever they be dressed, they comfort, nourish, and strengthen the bodie, procure bodily lust, and that with greediness.[2(pages780–1)]

"Eryngos" or "eringoes," *Eryngium*, spp., which are South American flowering plants, are "good for . . . people that have no delight or appetite to venery, nourishing and restoring . . . " when the roots are "condited or preserved with sugar."[2(page1000)] Other candied lust-inducers are "kernels of Fisticke nuts [*Pistacia vera*] condited, or made into comfits, with sugar,"[2(page1248)] and "Dates," *Phoenix dactylifera* and spp., which induce lust when prepared "by the cunning Confectioners."[2(page1334)]

Gerarde says that "Burre docke," *Arctium lappa*, with the rind removed from the stalk and the inner part "eaten rawe with salt and pepper, or boiled in the broth of fat meate . . . increaseth seed and stirreth up lust."[2(page665)] Though Cordelia mentions this plant rather as a weed, this is the plant that she means when she describes Lear as "crowned with . . . burdocks." (*King Lear*, IV.iv.3–4)

Love-in-idleness, *Viola tricolor*, plays a pivotal role in the plot of Shakespeare's *A Midsummer Night's Dream*.

> *Oberon.* Yet marked I where the bolt of Cupid fell.
> It fell upon a little western flower,
> Before milk-white, now purple with love's wound,
> And maidens call it love-in-idleness.
> Fetch me that flower, the herb I showed thee once.
> The juice of it on sleeping eyelids laid
> Will make or man or woman madly dote
> Upon the next live creature that it sees.
>
> (*Midsummer Night's Dream*, II.i.165–172; see
> also *Midsummer Night's Dream*, III.ii.102–104)

This plant was known to Elizabethans also as Harts ease, Pansies, Live in idelnes, Cull me to you, Three faces in a hood, and Kisse me ere I rise.[2(pages703–5 and appendix)] Its lust-inducing virtues probably are country folklore or Shakespeare's invention. None of the herbals mention lust-inducing properties for this plant. Gerarde says its "tough and slimie juice" has anti-syphilitic properties.[2(pages703–5)]

Plants which, prepared with wine and drunk, were thought by the sixteenth century English to induce lust are *Daucus carota* or "wilde carrot" roots,[2(page874)] *Galium verum* or "Ladies bedstraw" or "Maides haire" (roots),[2(page968)] and others. Lust-inducing properties were also attributed to boiled buds of *Helianthus annuus*, the sunflower,[2(pages612–4)] and to orchids, *Serapias* spp., *Cynorchis* spp., and *Orchis morio*. Orchids were also known as "stones" and "testicles;" and Gerarde says that "our age useth all the kindes of stones to stirre up venerie."[2(pages156–8, 169, 173–5)] Many plants were thought to procure lust in men only, "by increasing naturall seede;"[2(page754)] these were in much use by wives of the sixteenth century, for instance the cotton seed, *Gossypium* spp.

Poppy, Mandragora, and Other Sleep-inducing Drugs

Iago. Not poppy, nor mandragora,
Nor all the drowsy syrups of the world,
Shall ever medicine thee to that sweet sleep

Which thou owedst yesterday.

(*Othello*, III.iii.330–333)

Cleopatra. Give me to drink mandragora.

(*Antony and Cleopatra* I.v.4; see also
Romeo and Juliet IV.iii.47)

Langham says of the Poppy or Poppie, *Papaver* spp.
(opium),

Sleepe to cause, drink a spoonefull of syrupe of Poppy,
or anoint the temples with oyle of Poppy. Sleepe
to cause, take one spoonefull of white Poppy seede
with a little possiteale made with Violets, Strawberie
leaves, and Fiveleafe, and drink it warme when neede
is. [To prepare the spoonful:] Bruise 4. ounces of
white Poppy seede, but not that ripest, steepe them in
a pottel of rain water 24. hours, seethe it till the better
halfe be wasted, streine it, and to every pint put one
pound of Sugar, seethe it and skomme it, and keepe it
in a close glasse.[7(page508)]

And Gerarde states that of the "Garden poppie,"

Opium, or the harde juice of Poppie heads is strongest
of all: *Meconium* (which is the juice of the heads and
leaves) is weaker. Both of them any waies taken either
inwardly, or outwardly applied to the heade, provoke
sleepe. *Opium* somewhat too plentifully taken doth also
bring death.[2(page298)]

One of Langham's recipes for the use of Poppy indicates that Lady Macbeth may have drugged Duncan's grooms with Poppy. Langhan reports,

> Powder of white Poppie seede given to children in milke or possite drinke, or an alebrew, or rather with a Caudell of Almonds and hempe seede, causeth them to sleepe.[7(page507)]

Lady Macbeth's potion for the grooms was mixed in a posset, a warm drink of spiced milk curdled with ale or wine. (*Macbeth*, II.ii.5–8)

Gerarde says Mandrake or Mandragora, *Mandragora officinarum*, has a "drowsie and sleeping power," which is used by boiling the root in wine to drink, smelling the juice or the apples (fruit of the mandrake), or making a suppository of the juice.[2(page281)]

Additional "drowsy syrups" known to Elizabethans were oil of *Viola* spp. applied to the genitals,[2(page702)] the juice of tobacco, *Nicotiana* spp.,[2(pages285–7)] *Anethum graveolens* or dill boiled in "common oile,"[2(page878)] and others.

Nightshade: Inducing the Death-like Sleep

> *Friar Laurence.* And this distillèd liquor drink thou off,
> When presently through all thy veins shall run
> A cold and drowsy humor; for no pulse
> Shall keep his native progress, but surcease.
> No warmth, no breath, shall testify thou livest.

. . . .

And in this borrowed likeness of shrunk death
Thou shalt continue two and forty hours,
And then awake as from a pleasant sleep.

> (*Romeo and Juliet*, IV.i.94–98, 104–106)

The "sleeping Nightshade," *Atropa belladonna*, says
Gerarde, has a "pleasant and beautifull fruit," yet it is a
plant "furious and deadly."

> sleeping Nightshade . . . cometh very neere
> unto *Theophrastus* his *Mandragoras*, (which
> differeth from *Dioscorides* his *Mandragoras*) if
> there be a difference.
>
> This kinde of Nightshade causeth sleepe . . .
> [a small amount causes madness; moderate
> amounts cause a dead sleep] . . .
>
> . . . it bringeth such as have eaten thereof into a dead
> sleepe wherein many have died . . .
>
> The leaves hereof . . . imbibed or moistened in wine
> vinegar.[2(page270)]

Gerarde speaks of another herb that Shakespeare might
have had in mind when he described Friar Laurence's
potion; this potion might have been *Scirpus lacustris*,
the "Bull rush."

> The seede of the Bull rush is most soporiferous;
> and therefore the greater care must be had in the

administration thereof, least in provoking sleepe, you induce a drowsines, or deepe sleepe.[2(page32)]

In *Cymbeline*, Imogen's death-like sleep may have been induced by the sleeping Nightshade or the Bull rush. The Queen, says the physician Cornelius, will see this drug appear to kill cats and dogs; but when she uses it on humans, it will only create a dead sleep. (*Cymbeline*, I.v.33–42) Gerarde mentions one other drug that might fit this description, *Doronicum* spp.

> Leopards bane . . . killeth Panthers, swine, wolves . . . this herbe or the root thereof is not deadly to man, but to divers beasts onely . . . That this *Aconite* killeth dogs, it is very certaine and founde out by triall.[2(pages619–22)]

Henbane: the Death of Hamlet's Father

Hamlet's father was poisoned with "hebenon." It is likely that this "hebenon" was henbane, *Hyoscyamus* spp., even though Shakespeare's description of the symptoms does not exactly coincide with those discussed in any herbal of the time.

> *Ghost.* ... Sleeping within my orchard,
> My custom always of the afternoon,
> Upon my secure hour thy uncle stole

With juice of cursèd hebenon in a vial,
And in the porches of my ears did pour
The leperous distillment, whose effect
Holds such an enmity with blood of man
That swift as quicksilver it courses through
The natural gates and alleys of the body,
And with a sudden vigor it doth posset
And curd, like eager droppings into milk,
The thin and wholesome blood. So did it mine,
And a most instant tetter barked about,
Most lazarlike, with vile and loathsome crust,
All my smooth body.

(*Hamlet*, I.v.59–73)

The sixteenth century English believed that medicinal drugs could reach the rest of the body through the ears. Banckes mentions two drugs that can treat the brain and the stomach by means of "juice dropped in the ears of a man."[3(pages17, 31)] Langham says that to "wash the . . . eares" with henbane seethed in wine will bring sleep.[7(page310)]

Henbane, also called Henbell, *Symphoniaca*, and jusquiamus,[2(appendices)] was thought to have penetrating powers; medicinally, one would "apply it to sores that rot at the bone."[7(page308)] Symptoms of henbane poisoning in the herbals are similar but not identical to those of hebenon in *Hamlet*. Gerarde says it produces a sleep that "is deadly to the partie"[2(page284)] when ingested. It is indeed possible that Shakespeare misread Langham's statement that "Scabs, pockes, and Leapry, take up the fume of the seede to the grieved parte,"[7](page309) leading to the statement of symptoms that Hamlet's father's ghost described (above).

Banquo may have spoken of henbane[16] when he said of the vision of the Weird Sisters:

> *Banquo.* Were such things here as we do
>   speak about?
> Or have we eaten on the insane root
> That takes the reason prisoner?
>
>   (*Macbeth*, I.iii.83–85)

Langham says of henbane, "Anoint thy temples with the juice, and thou shalt see mervailes in thy sleepe."[7](page308) Henbane is the only drug I've found in the herbals that could be described as "insane;" and the "juice" could be from the root, presumably.

Aconite

> *King Henry.* ... though it do work as strong
> As aconitum . . .
>
>   (*2 Henry IV*, IV.iv.47–48)

Gerarde differentiates between "Aconite or Woolfes bane . . . surnamed *Valdensis*," and "*Napellus*, or Munckes hoode, which is likewise named *Thora*."[2](page818) He states that all aconites are "deadly to man, likewise to all other living creatures."[2](page822) Langham says of "Monkshood . . . They are strong poyson to be taken inward."[7](page405)

Aconites were also described as arrow and sword poisons.

Arrow and Sword Poisons

> *Laertes.* And for that purpose I'll anoint
>   my sword.
> I bought an unction of a mountebank
> So mortal that but dip a knife in it,
> Where it draws blood no cataplasm so rare,
> Collected from all simples that have virtue
> Under the moon, can save the thing from death
> That is but scratched withal. I'll touch my point
> With this contagion, that if I gall him slightly,
> It may be death.
>
>   (*Hamlet*, IV.vii.141–149)

> *Laertes.* No medicine in the world can do
>   thee good,
> In thee there is not half an hour of life.
>
>   (*Hamlet*, V.ii.325–326)

> *Hamlet.* Oh, I die, Horatio,
> The potent poison quite o'ercrows my spirit.
>
>   (*Hamlet*, V.ii.363–364)

Hamlet dies within "half an hour" after being poisoned probably with Aconite or Woolfes bane. Gerarde says of non-yellow Woolfes banes that "if a man . . . be wounded with an arrowe or other instrument dipped in the juice heareof, [he] doth die within halfe an hower after remedilesse."[2(page818)]

Gerarde describes the symptoms of *oral* ingestion of Aconite arrow poison as conceivably similar to the symptoms of the sword poison that "o'ercrows" Hamlet:

> The symptomes that followe those that do eate of these deadly herbes are these; their lips and toongs swell foorthwith, their eies hang out, their thighes are stiffe, and their wits are taken from them . . . if the points of darts or arrowes be touched with the same, it bringeth deadly hurt to those that be wounded therewith.[2(page824)]

Elizabethan England's herbalists also knew of the South American arrow poisons. Monardes describes cannibal Indians who

> have kylled with their arrowes which are poysoned with these venemous hearbes, an infinite number of Spaniardes. ... [the victim's] fleshe is harde . . . the hearbe which they shoote withall, for that it maketh them to dye by madnesse.[8(page69)]

Deadly Poison with Delayed Effect

> *Cornelius.* ... She did confess she had
> For you a mortal mineral, which, being took,
> Should by the minute feed on life and lingering
> By inches waste you . . .
>   (*Cymbeline*, V.v.49–52)

The symptoms described by Cornelius might be those of Speare Crowfoote or Banewoort, whose victims "have died with great torment."[2](page815) These poisons are from *Atropa belladonna* and some species of *Ranunculus*. (Other references to deadly poisons with delayed effects can be found at *Tempest*, III.iii.104–106 and *King Lear*, V.iii.95–96.)

Winter Woolfes Bane: Hot and Dry Death

It is very possible that Shakespeare's King John was poisoned with Winter Woolfes bane or small yellowe Woolfes bane, *Eranthis hyemalis*.

> *Hubert.* The King, I fear, is poisoned by a monk.
> I left him almost speechless. ...
> . . . .
> *Bastard.* How did he take it? Who did taste
>   to him?
> *Hubert.* A monk, I tell you, a resolvèd villain,
> Whose bowels suddenly burst out. The King
> Yet speaks and peradventure may recover.
>
>   (*King John*, V.vi.23–24, 28–31)

> *Pembroke.* ... the burning quality
> Of that fell poison . . .
> *Prince Henry.* Doth he still rage?
>
>   (*King John*, V.vii.8–9, 11)

The burning quality of Gerarde's Winter Woolfes bane comes closest to this characteristic among Elizabethan poisons. "We have great quantities of it in our London gardens. … This herbe is counted to be very dangerous and deadly: hot & drie in the fourth degree."[2(pages818–9)] An herb is hot in the fourth degree, says Turner, if it "be so hot as it can be." These "burn and … fret inward.[17]

Hemlocke and Darnell

> *Cordelia.* Alack, 'tis he. Why, he was met
>   even now
> As mad as the vexed sea, singing aloud,
> Crowned with …
> … hemlock …
> Darnel, and all the idle weeds that grow.
>
>   (*King Lear*, IV.iv.1–5)

> *Burgundy.* … Her fallow leas
> The darnel, hemlock …
> Doth root upon while that the colter rusts.
>
>   (*Henry V*, V.ii.44–46)

> *3. Witch.* Root of hemlock digged i' the dark.
>
>   (*Macbeth*, IV.i.25)

Shakespeare refers to both *Cicuta virosa*, the water hemlock, and to *Conium maculatum*, the poison hemlock of Socrates. These plants are both members of the parsley family, the Umbelliferae. Both are weeds and both are poisonous. *Cicuta virosa* grows at the edges of rivers and ditches in Great Britain. *Conium maculatum* grows wild among ruins and on hedge banks and the borders of fields. It has a long tap root and may therefore be the particular hemlock used by the witches in *Macbeth*.

The Elizabethan English differentiated between water hemlocks and the hemlock of Socrates, but they believed the pharmacological properties to be identical. Gerarde says that the water hemlock's "temperature and faculties are answerable to the Common Hemlocke." Both were known to have a noxious odor and to be very poisonous. Interestingly, Gerarde's *cicuta* or herbe Bennet is *Conium maculatum*.[18] Gerarde's cicutaria or "the wilde and water hemlocks" is *Cicuta virosa* and other species. Gerarde says that the leaf of Hemlocke

> is a very evil, dangerous, hurtfull, and poisonous herbe, insomuch that whosoever taketh of it into his body dieth remedilesse . . . but being drunke with wine the poison is with greater speede carried to the hart, by reason whereof it killeth presently.[2(page904)]

Langham says of Hemlocke, "The juice is a strong poyson."[7(page305)]

Gerarde also says of Hemlocke, that it "groweth plentifully about towne wals and villages in shadowy places, and fat soiles neere ditches,"[2(page903)] and his wood-cut drawing of the Hemlocke is indeed fat. This information suggests that the ghost of Hamlet's father perhaps was speaking of Hemlocke when he said,

> *Ghost.* And duller shouldst thou be than the
> fat weed
> That roots itself in ease on Lethe warf
> Wouldst thou not stir in this.
>
> (*Hamlet*, I.v.32–34)

Langham says of Darnell, *Lolium* spp., "Put it into Ale or Beere, it causeth drunkennes, and troubleth the braine."[7(page188)] Gerarde says it is only poisonous in that it "hurteth the eies and maketh them dim."[2(page72)]

Ratsbane

There are numerous references to rat poisons in the plays. For instance,

> *Claudio.* ... Our natures do pursue,
> Like rats that ravin down their proper bane,
> A thirsty evil, and when we drink we die.
>
> (*Measure for Measure*, I.ii.132–134)

> *Shepherd.* ... I would the milk
> Thy mother gave thee when thou suck'dst
> her breast
> Had been a little ratsbane for thy sake!
>
> (*1 Henry VI*, V.iv.27–29; see also *2 Henry IV*,
> I.ii.46–48; *King Lear*, III.iv.51–56)

Bankes says that powdered *Helleborus niger* "will destroy and slay rats."[3(page28)] Gerarde reports that *Veratrum album*, known to Elizabethans as white Hellebor, Nieswoort, Lingwoort, and Roote neesing, "the roote given to drinke in the waight of two pence . . . killeth mice and rattes being made up with honie and flower of wheate."[2(page357)]

Mosses and Mistletoes

> *Tamora.* The trees, though summer, yet forlorn and
>   lean,
> O'ercome with moss and baleful mistletoe.
>
>   (*Titus Andronicus*, II.iii.94–95)

A poisonous glue, known to Elizabethans as *Ixia* or Birdlime, was made from the berries of the Misseltoe, or Misteltoe, or Missell. This is *Viscum album* and *Loranthus* spp. Gerarde says:

> This birdlime inwardly taken is mortall, and bringeth most greevous accidents, the toong is inflamed and swolne, the minde is distraughted, the strength of the hart and wits faile.[2(pages1168–70)]

He further adds that the Mosse Ferne, *Polypodium dryopteris*, "hath in the roote a harsh or choking taste, and a mortifying qualitie, and therefore it taketh away haires."[2(page974)] Most likely, though, Shakespeare meant by "moss" specifically the moss of trees, which was supposed to have soporific qualities.[2(page 1370)]

Yew

> *Scroop.* Thy very beadsmen learn to bend
>   their bows
> Of double-fatal yew against thy state.
>
> > (*Richard II*, III.ii.116–117)

> *3. Witch.* ... and slips of yew
> Slivered in the moon's eclipse.
>
> > (*Macbeth*, IV.i.27–28)

Gerarde says of the yew, *Taxus* spp., that it is reported that it

> is of a venemous qualitie, and against mans nature. Dioscorides writeth, and generally all that heretofore have dealt in the facultie of herbarisme, that the Yew tree is very venemous to be taken inwardly, and that if any do sleepe under the shadow thereof, it causeth sicknes, and oftentimes death. Moreover, they say that the fruite thereof being eaten, is not onely dangerous unto man and deadly . . . All which I dare boldly affirme, is altogither untrue. For when I was yoong and went to schoole, divers of my schoole fellowes and likewise my selfe did eate our fils of the berries of this tree, and have not onely slept under the shadow thereof, but among the branches also,

without any hurt at all, and that not one time, but many times.[2(page1188)]

Mushrooms

Prospero. ... and you whose pastime
Is to make midnight mushrooms that rejoice
To hear the solemn curfew . . .

    (*Tempest*, V.i.38–40)

Gerarde says of "Mushrums" that "most of them do suffocate and strangle the eater."[2(page1386)] He quotes from Virgil's "first book of Georgickes" a passage in translation about "up rotten Mushrums be growne" in the "night."[2(page1387)] Elsewhere he says that mushrooms are "venemous and deadly . . . [and] may procure untimely death."[2(page274)]

Other Deadly Poisons

Apothecary. ... Put this in any liquid thing
    you will,
And drink it off, and if you had the strength
Of twenty men, it would dispatch you straight.

    (*Romeo and Juliet*, V.i.77–79)

Although there is no way with certainty to identify the poison described here that Romeo drinks, because the description is insufficient, there are several deadly poisons discussed by Gerarde in addition to those already mentioned. Herbe Christopher or Aconitum bacciferum (*Actaea spicata, Osmunda regalis*), says Gerarde, is as "deadly and remedilesse" as Ratsbane.[2(page829)] And the Ash tree, *Fraxinus* spp., "the shivers or small peeces thereof . . . being drunke, are saide to be pernicious and deadly."[2(page1289)]

The Death of Hamlet's Mother

King Claudius prepares a poison for Hamlet.

> *King.* The King shall drink to Hamlet's
>   better breath,
> And in the cup a union shall he throw
> Richer than that which four successive kings
> In Denmark's crown have worn.
>
>   (*Hamlet*, V.ii.282–285)

But contrary to his intentions, his Queen drinks from the chalice. It is interesting to note the use of the word "union" for pill. Another usage of the time was "pearles" in which Monardes recommended dosages, "prepared of everie one the waight of twelve pence."[8(page120)]

12

The Politician Who
Loved Shakespeare

Politicians often quote Shakespeare, but none have done it in so meaningful a way as Senator Robert F. Kennedy. He had begun reading Shakespeare's plays late in life and took their deep insights to heart. Perhaps also he could see "Shakespearean" aspects of the role he was now playing in American politics. After the assassination of his brother, President John F. Kennedy, in 1963, he was elected US Senator in 1964 and was widely viewed as someone who might replace President Lyndon Johnson in 1968. The assassination of his brother, his own popularity, and Johnson's jealousy had some of the grandeur and drama of a Shakespearean play.

At the same time, Kennedy was developing a passion for literature for the first time in his life. Many people have said that he was using literature to try to make sense of the assassination of his brother. He read

Shakespeare's plays[1,2] and many other works of literature[1,3,4], even the book that Shakespeare used as a source for background information for his plays about ancient Rome, Plutarch's *Lives*.[1]

Kennedy memorized long passages and quoted Shakespeare in conversations, speeches, and letters.[5,6] His daughter, Kathleen Kennedy Townsend, said that she could hear him listening to recordings of Shakespeare while he did sit-ups in the morning,[7] and he was also reported to have listened to recordings of Shakespeare's plays while shaving.[2] There was a Kennedy family story of him surpassing Richard Burton in an informal "Shakespeare reciting contest in front of Elizabeth Taylor."[7]

Quoting *Romeo and Juliet*: "Take him and cut him out in little stars"

He spoke to the Democratic National Convention in Atlantic City, NJ in 1964 to introduce a film about the late President John Kennedy. He set aside his prepared speech and spoke extemporaneously,[5] quoting Juliet's soliloquy from Shakespeare's *Romeo and Juliet*:

> When I think of President Kennedy, I think of what
>   Shakespeare said in *Romeo and Juliet*:
>
> When he shall die
> Take him and cut him out in little stars
> And he will make the face of heaven so fine

That all the world will be in love with night,
And pay no worship to the garish sun.

(*Romeo and Juliet*, III.ii.21–25)[5]

Quoting *Henry IV, Part II*: "For this they . . . invest their sons"

In a discussion with the poet Robert Lowell, Kennedy took down a volume of Shakespeare's plays and read aloud a section of the king's deathbed speech in *Henry IV, Part II*, in order to illustrate a point about his own father[1]:

> For this the foolish overcareful fathers
> Have broke their sleep with thoughts, their brains
>   with care,
> Their bones with industry.
> For this they have engrossed and pilèd up
> The cankered heaps of strange-achievèd gold.
> For this they have been thoughtful to invest
> Their sons with arts and martial exercises.
>
> (*2 Henry IV*, IV.v.68–74)[8]

He was illustrating how his own father had built up wealth for his descendants. He then quoted the king saying that the younger generation had an easy time because:

> . . . for what in me was purchased
> Falls upon thee in a more fairer sort . . .
>
> (*2 Henry IV*, IV.v.200–201)[8]

Quoting *Henry V*: "We few, we happy few, we band of brothers"

Kennedy frequently quoted the "St. Crispin's Day Speech" from Shakespeare's *Henry V*, in which the king exhorts his troops before the Battle of Agincourt. The battle took place during the Hundred Years' War, on October 25, 1415, which happened to be the feast day for the twin martyred saints, Crispin and Crispian:

> This story shall the good man teach his son,
> And Crispin Crispian shall ne'er go by,
> From this day to the ending of the world,
> But we in it shall be remembered –
> We few, we happy few, we band of brothers.
> For he today that sheds his blood with me
> Shall be my brother. Be he ne'er so vile,
> This day shall gentle his condition.
> And gentlemen in England now abed
> Shall think themselves accursed they were
>   not here,
> And hold their manhoods cheap whiles
>   any speaks
> That fought with us upon Saint Crispin's Day.
>
> (*Henry V*, IV.iii.60–67)[8]

Kathleen Kennedy Townshend says he "often recited the St. Crispian [*sic*] Day speech. Among his friends, and with us children as we walked the grounds at Hickory Hill [their home] or in the woods nearby."[9]

She recalled, "I remember walking with my father one cool evening. It was just the two of us at twilight, and the stars were just starting to come out. The President had died a few months before. My father was telling me how [President Kennedy had] tried to create the best administration, what an extraordinary group of people had worked in that effort, and how special that time had been. He then quoted, as we walked, the Crispian [*sic*] Day speech . . . " beginning with "This story shall the good man tell [*sic*] his son . . . "[7]

During a strenuous seven-mile climb with his family and other adults coming out of the Grand Canyon in 1967, one of the adults suggested that they turn back. Kennedy replied by quoting from the St. Crispin's Day speech, "We few, we happy few, we band of brothers. For he today that sheds his blood with me shall be my brother . . . " His wife then urged him, "Say the whole thing," and he did so, and then quoted the entire speech a second time later that day, when the group was again flagging.[10,11]

He also used the phrase, "We few, we happy few, we band of brothers," on a memento picture frame. In 1965, he and seven other men were the first to climb to the peak of the 14,000-foot Mount Kennedy in the Canadian Yukon, which had recently been named for President Kennedy. He gave each climber a photograph from the climb, with "We few, we happy few, we band of brothers" engraved on the metal picture frame.[12]

Reading *Coriolanus*

Coriolanus is said to be Shakespeare's most political play.[13] It has a message for politicians: Listen to the citizens, and do not scorn the common people among those you would govern. One of Kennedy's top aides once gave him a copy of *Coriolanus,* saying, "You *have* to read *this* one."[12] It may seem like a strange reading recommendation, since Kennedy probably had the greatest empathy of any politician for ordinary citizens and disadvantaged people. The aide probably wanted Kennedy to be conscious of the risk posed by his opponents who were portraying him as a "ruthless" politician focused only on becoming President.

His Widespread Reading and his Commonplace Book

After his brother's assassination, Robert Kennedy went through a very introspective period, began to take long meditative walks, and began to read intensively.[3] He read books by Albert Camus, Ralph Waldo Emerson, the ancient Greek historians Herodotus and Thucydides, and the ancient Greek playwrights Aeschylus, Euripides, and Sophocles.[3,4] He read *The Greek Way* and several other books by Edith Hamilton.[3,4] He received reading recommendations from Jacqueline Kennedy, the poet Robert Lowell, and others.[1,3] For a while, one of his senior aides recommended a new book every week.[12] He always had a book of literature in his briefcase along with the office papers he was taking home to work on.[12]

He selected quotations from his reading by underlining or bracketing them in pencil in the books,[3,12] and his staff typed them on pages for a 6-inch loose-leaf notebook containing quotations.[12] He also wrote some of the same quotations by hand on 3 × 5 cards that he carried in his shirt pocket with a rubber band around them, and he reviewed them in the minutes before delivering a speech.[12] He quoted liberally from them, especially during question-and-answer sessions with younger audiences.[12]

Robert Kennedy's strong interest in Shakespeare in these years communicated that he was thinking about timeless issues. It showed that he recognized the deep currents flowing through western culture and their influence on the societal problems of the times. It communicated his respect for the wisdom that can be found in Shakespeare's writing.

13

Mr. Siegel Was King Lear

By the time I entered medical school, I had already read Shakespeare's *King Lear* three times; in retrospect, even then I was still too young to understand it. Although I saw it as a story about old age and retirement, I was unable to see that it is Shakespeare's deepest and most penetrating analysis of interactions between parents and their adult children.

I lived near the medical school in a fourth-floor, rent-controlled apartment in a decaying neighborhood. The floors of the apartment sloped. The living room had a hot steam pipe in a corner that was supposed to help with the heating. The interior walls were thin, and I could hear some of my neighbors. The two windows on the fire escape had metal gates and padlocks, and a padlock key hung on a hook nearby.

On my move-in day, I had knocked next door and introduced myself to the elderly Hungarian immigrants who lived there, Mr. and Mrs. Siegel. Mr. Siegel was lively, spry, and spoke almost perfect English. Mrs. Siegel seemed older than her husband and her English was difficult to understand. She was a big woman, and it seemed that she may have been very beautiful when she was younger. Now she was tall and weak, always in a housecoat. I could hear her struggling to get to the door when anyone knocked. I never saw her leave her apartment.

A few days after I moved in, Mr. Siegel knocked on my door to bring me a plate of warm food. When he said it was "from" Mrs. Siegel, he may have meant that the "gift" was from her, since I think he had probably cooked it himself because Mrs. Siegel was probably too weak to stand at the stove. Looking back, I see the plate of food as a request for friendship.

I knocked on their door the next day to thank them. As we talked, Mr. Siegel proudly told me that they had two daughters who lived in large houses in the suburbs with their spouses and children. I thought he was trying to say that they were not just an old couple living alone in an old building on a decaying street, but that they were parents of successful daughters. However, during the year I lived there, I never saw the daughters visit, either alone or with the grandchildren.

I moved away the next year to a newly constructed high-rise, but I often walked down that street near the medical school. Sometimes I ran into Mr. Siegel on the street. He would ask me how my studies were going, and I would ask how he and Mrs. Siegel were doing. When I ran into him a year and a half later, he told me that Mrs. Siegel had died.

I didn't see Mr. Siegel again until another year had passed. He introduced me to the people he was walking with, Vietnamese immigrants to whom he was teaching English. He added that he also gave them advice about how to get along in the US.

And then I forgot about him until decades later. It was then that I remembered Mr. Siegel and his two daughters who never visited, and I realized that Mr. Siegel's sorrow had been in plain sight.

I thought about King Lear, who had retired and left his kingdom to the oldest two of his three adult daughters, swayed by their exaggerated descriptions of their love for him. He was soon thrown out of the castle into a stormy landscape, first by one daughter and then by another. Many years ago, a *New Yorker* cartoon showed King Lear raging against the storm, as two children walk by and one says, "Don't remind him it's Father's Day."

I realized that Mr. Siegel *was* King Lear, in the way that Shakespeare truly saw King Lear. Shakespeare wrote *King Lear* about old age but also about the timeless estrangement of adult children from their parents.

Perhaps Shakespeare had had similar experiences. Late in his life, Shakespeare had acquired a sizeable estate due to successful real estate and agricultural investments. When he died in 1616 at age 52, he left to his oldest daughter Susanna, born in 1583, three houses in Stratford, an apartment in London, and various lands around Stratford. He left only some money to his other daughter, Judith, born in 1585. The imbalance in his bequests suggests that he, too, may have been King Lear.

Years ago, I was too young to recognize the sorrow of "old" Mr. Siegel. Now, more than 50 years later, I am even older than Mr. Siegel was then – and now I understand.

14

Shakespeare's Bilingual Play

Shakespeare's play *Henry V*[1] tells the story of the Hundred Years' War between England and France (1337–1453). Although the play was written for English audiences, many of its French characters speak some lines in French during seven of the nine scenes in which they appear.[2] In two other Shakespeare plays about wars between England and France (*Henry VI Part I* and *King John*), the French characters speak only English.

In *Henry* V, some French is spoken in discussions between the French leaders, in discussions between French soldiers, in an English lesson conducted mainly in French for the French princess, and in a bilingual courtship between King Henry and the French princess. There are two additional scenes in which English soldiers use some French phrases.

Shakespeare may have made his French characters speak the French language to make them more realistic. The opening of the play and each of the acts have

"Prologues" in which Shakespeare showed that he was thinking about realism and the difficulty of portraying a war on a stage. In the prologue to the play, he asks, "Can this cockpit hold the vasty fields of France? . . . Think when we talk of horses that you see them . . . " (*Henry V*, Prologue.11–12;26), and in the Prologue to Act III he says to the audience, "Work, work your thoughts, and therein see a siege" (*Henry V*, III.Prologue.25).

In modern times, when plays have lines in another language, there may be electronic "surtitles" with English translations, but these were not available to Shakespeare. Theoretically his theater company could have used placards with English translations, but there is no evidence that they did so.

The French dialogue in *Henry V* strongly suggests that some people in the audience understood French. The French lines are sometimes complex; one character states a complex French proverb: *"Le chien est retourné à son propre vomissement, et la truie lavée au bourbier"* [*Henry V*, III.vii.68–69], meaning "The dog returned to his own vomit and the sow bathed in a pool of mud." Shakespeare would not have expected these lines to be successful unless he knew that some of his audience understood French.

Once Shakespeare had decided to create a bilingual play, he apparently decided to take advantage of its ability to provide comic relief. In an English lesson for the French princess, pronunciation mistakes result in bawdy misunderstandings and bilingual puns. In Shakespeare's time, perhaps even Londoners who could not speak French may have been familiar with French obscenities. But Shakespeare also included the English lesson in order to make the observation that mispronounced words in one language can mean something embarrassing in another language. When the princess asks how to say "elbow," "neck," "chin," "foot," and "gown" in English, either she or her teacher mispronounces the English words (*"bilbow," "nick," "sin," "foot," "coun"*), two of which (*"bilbow"* and *"nick"*) are obscenities in Elizabethan English, and two others (*"foot"* and *"coun"*) were obscene in French (*Henry V,* III:iv:1–54). The princess is shocked by the words she has been taught, and she says, *"Je ne voudrais prononcer ces mots devant les seigneurs de France pour tout le monde"* ("I would not for all the world want to pronounce these words in front of the lords of France") (*Henry V,* III.iv.58–59).

Shakespeare used a stage technique to provide some indirect translations. In some scenes, he had characters restate the French lines in English. For instance, when the princess says, *"Les langues des hommes sont pleines de trumperies,"* King Henry replies, "What says she . . . ? That the tongues of men are full of deceits?" (*Henry V,* V.ii.118–121), and this functions as a translation for those in the audience who could not understand French.

We do not actually know whether Shakespeare ever formally studied French, and it is doubtful whether he had ever travelled to France. We don't even know whether

Shakespeare wrote the French lines himself or whether he had help. However, there were many French Huguenot expatriates living in London at that time, from whom Shakespeare may have learned some French; in fact, he lodged with one Huguenot family a few years after he wrote *Henry V*. The bawdy bilingual puns are consistent with examples of Shakespeare's bawdy humor in English in some of his other plays, and these suggest that he himself wrote the baudy French lines.

Shakespeare also harvests another kind of bilingual humor when the English soldier, Pistol, misunderstands the pleas of a captured French soldier. The French soldier pleads *"Seigneur Dieu"* ("Lord God"), which Pistol thinks is a French name "Signieur Dew." He thinks that *"moi"* is a unit of currency, that *"bras"* for "arm" means "brass," and that *"pardonnez moi"* means "a ton of moys" (*Henry V*, IV.iv.6–22). Pistol also speaks a nonsense phrase that he thinks sounds like French (*Henry V*, IV.iv.4).

In this play, English soldiers incorrectly use the French word *"rendezvous"* (*Henry V*, II.i.17–18) and mispronounce *"couper la gorge"* ("cut his throat") as "couple a gorge" (*Henry V*, II.i.73–75). When the disguised English King Henry says his name is "Harry le Roy" (*Henry V*, IV.i.49), the English soldier does not recognize it as French for "Henry the King," and asks if it is a Cornish name.

Even audience members who could not understand French can enjoy the play, just as readers today can enjoy Tolstoy's *War and Peace*, of which 2% was in French in the original Russian version, and the French has been retained in many English editions. By keeping spoken French in his dialog, Shakespeare achieved greater realism than he would have had if the enemy soldiers and leaders had spoken on stage only in heavily accented English.

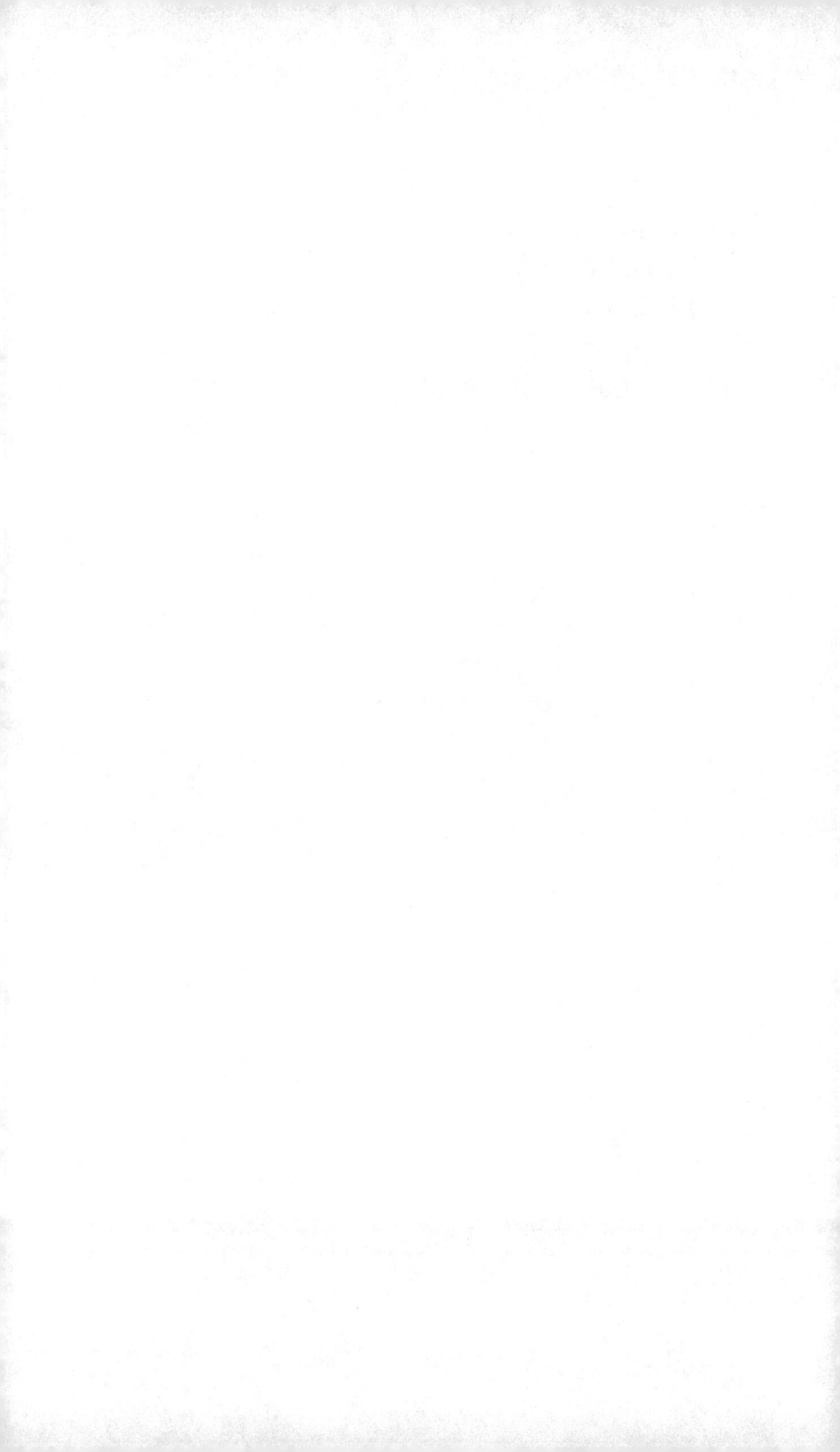

15

Shakespeare and Memory

Shakespeare wrote for the stage, and he could not have imagined the way his writings would someday be memorized and quoted in classrooms, or the way phrases from his writings and some words that he created would become parts of ordinary speech.

He wrote the plays for actors, not readers. He wrote for his actors to make a living, and for the company to remain solvent. His plays were performed during his lifetime, but some of his best plays were not published during his lifetime.

Shakespeare seems to have taken for granted that actors memorize lines. In *A Midsummer Night's Dream*, the workmen-actors are assigned to learn their lines "by tomorrow night" (*Midsummer Night's Dream*, I.ii.101–103),[1] although one of them, Snug, mentions that "I am slow of study." (*Midsummer Night's Dream*, I.ii.69) But in *Hamlet*, when Hamlet gives a fairly long critique of the characteristics of good and bad actors, and how actors should deliver their lines (*Hamlet*, III.ii.1–53), he makes no mention of the process of memorizing the lines.

When Shakespeare does use the word "memorize" in his plays, he uses it with a different meaning than our modern usage. In Elizabethan English, "memorize" (or sometimes spelled "memorise"[2]) meant "memorialize." Shakespeare only used the word twice (*Henry VIII*, III:ii:52; *Macbeth* I:ii:40).[2]

Shakespeare used the word "memorial" four times, meaning something that reminds us to remember, such as a line in a poem (*Sonnet* 74), a statue (*Troilus and Cressida*, V.1.59–60; *Twelfth Night*, III.iii.23), or the glove of a beloved (*Troilus and Cressida*, V.ii.79–80).

Shakespeare used the word "memory" 58 times and "memories" 3 times. In the plays, "memory" sometimes means a thing that reminds us of bad times, for instance when Lear's daughter Cordelia says "These weeds are memories of those worser hours" (*King Lear*, IV.vii.7). Shakespeare particularly liked to talk about "memory" in the Sonnets (used 8 times), usually referring to the mental place where a record of a person's beauty or love is preserved, even after the person's beauty has diminished or the person has died. He says that memory is a better place to store the record than a mere notebook ("tables" in Elizabethan usage) (*Sonnet* 122).

Nevertheless, even though he saw memory as better than a notebook, he also referred to memory as a kind of notebook to write in. He used the Elizabethan word for a notebook, "table" (related to the word "tablet"). After the ghost of Hamlet's father tells him, "Remember me" (*Hamlet*, I.v.91), Hamlet refers to "the table of my memory" in which events are "copied," and he resolves to remove all other, trivial items from it:

> Yea, from the table of my memory
> I'll wipe away all trivial fond records,
> All saws of books, all forms, all pressures past,
> That youth and observation copied there,
> And thy commandment all alone shall live
> Within the book and volume of my brain,
> Unmixed with baser matter.
>
> (*Hamlet*, I.v.98–104)

In *Henry IV, Part II*, the archbishop says that the king will clear his "tables" of "memory":

> And therefore will he wipe his tables clean,
> And keep no telltale to his memory
> That may repeat and history his loss
> To new remembrance.
>
> (*2 Henry IV*, IV.i.201–204)

In *Henry VI, Part I*, Richard Plantagenet refers to memory as a book:

> I'll note you in my book of memory
> To scourge you for this apprehension.
>
> (*1 Henry VI*, II.iv.101–102)

The concept of memory as a notebook or tablet derives from ancient Greek philosophy. Aristotle, for instance, described the mind as "a blank writing-tablet with a capacity of receiving written characters."[3]

In *Hamlet*, Polonius exhorts Laertes with the now-famous list of precepts, and urges him to "character," i.e. to inscribe, the precepts in memory:

> And these few precepts in thy memory
> Look thou character.
>
> (*Hamlet*, I.iii.58–59)

Yet Shakespeare knew something about the anatomy of the brain. He wrote that ideas are created "in the ventricle of memory, nourished in the womb of pia mater, and delivered upon the mellowing of occasion." (*Love's Labor's Lost*, IV.ii.72–74) Here, he was saying that he believed memory is located in one of the ventricles, the spaces within the brain that contain cerebrospinal fluid, and in the pia mater, which is the inner lining of the membrane surrounding the brain and spinal cord. He was saying that ideas are stored there until the right occasion occurs for them to be "delivered."

Compared to modern authors, Shakespeare had a more limited number of metaphors available to describe how memory works. In modern times, memory is often said to be like an electronic recording, a computer, or a case of photographic slides, from which one takes out one memory at a time and looks at it. None of these concepts were available, of course, for Shakespeare to use as metaphors for memory.

Historical Moments

16

Justice Souter

Supreme Court Justice David Souter announced plans to retire from the Court in spring 2009. When I was a freshman at Harvard College in 1965–1966, Souter was a law student and served as a proctor for undergraduates in my dormitory, Straus Hall, but not for the students in the entry I lived in.

My roommates and I had a suite of rooms in C entry, separated by a sealed fire door from Souter's suite, which was in B entry. Any time our voices were raised, Souter could hear us through the fire door, and we could hear Souter sometimes. At least one time—and probably more often—he came over to our rooms to ask us to be quiet. One Saturday after midnight, Souter left his steady girlfriend, an Emmanuel College student, for a few minutes, exited his entry, walked up the stairs in our entryway, and asked us to keep the noise down. He said in a friendly way, "I am sitting with my date and I am just about to say 'My dear . . . ' and then 'Oh shit!' comes through the fire door." We did also have conversations with him about other topics besides noise.

In March, when rowing practice was scheduled throughout spring break, I was thinking about leaving the rowing team so that I could go home on spring break to see the cherry blossoms in Washington, DC where I lived. Souter came over to our suite to ask us what we were all doing for spring break. When he heard my possible plans, he strongly urged me to stay in Cambridge for rowing practice, saying, "Throughout your life, how many opportunities will you have to see the cherry blossoms, and how many opportunities will you have to row on crew?"

Souter always wore a white shirt, tie, and sport coat, and never wore an overcoat even in the middle of winter, at least on sunny days. Wearing a tweed sport coat and tie, he would wrap his Oxford scarf (from his years as a Rhodes Scholar) around his neck and, with his hands in his pockets, would set off along the shoveled paths between the mounds of snow.

I first learned that Souter had been appointed to the U.S. Supreme Court in 1990 when I suddenly heard his voice on my car radio while I was driving home from work. I had turned on the radio in the middle of an interview. I immediately recognized his voice after 24 years, even before I heard the announcer say his name; after all, I had heard that voice through the fire door every day for a year when I was a college freshman.

Soon afterwards, I wrote to congratulate him; about a year later I received a three-page handwritten reply. He said that he had saved all of his correspondence received during his first year on the Supreme Court and had taken it to his mother's farm in New Hampshire to answer after the end of the session.

After the announcement of his retirement, the news media praised his wisdom, his fairness, and his Thoreau-like dedication to a life free of unnecessary distractions.

17

Harvard Scholars in English

I recently came across the book, *Harvard Scholars in English, 1890–1990*,[1] a collection of biographical sketches of 21 professors of English who taught at Harvard University. In the late 1960s I was an enthusiastic Harvard undergraduate concentrating in English, but I was surprised now to learn so much about the English Department of those years.

For instance, Professor Douglas Bush was known among the faculty for his extraordinary memory. He had memorized the approximately 11,000 lines of Milton's *Paradise Lost* and recited them silently to himself to occupy his time on a train journey to Chicago.

I was surprised to learn that Professor John M. Bullitt, the first Master of the newly created Quincy House,[2] had been a subject in the Harvard Grant Study,[3] a renowned longitudinal study of normal development in 268 Harvard students. The participants entered the study as college sophomores and were followed with physical, psychological, and social evaluations throughout their lives. Participants were anonymous, but Professor Bullitt revealed his role and told his colleagues, "When they follow us out to our later years, they will get a shock." At the peak of his own career, he resigned his mastership of Quincy House and took a leave of absence from teaching to join the Peace Corps for two years in Bolivia.

The senior editor of this book was Walter Jackson Bate, also a noted professor in the English Department. He gave an extremely popular course called "The Age of Johnson," in which he seemed almost to transform into the famous Dr. Johnson during his lectures.

While I was caught up in this nostalgia, I took a look at the English course offerings in the four course catalogs from my years at Harvard. When I was a student, I had not known that I would still have these 44 years after I graduated. I had written notes in them during the "shopping period" for classes, a unique Harvard process allowing students to choose their classes by trying them out (a process that was officially eliminated in 2020[4]) – including my notation that a tutor in Winthrop House had said that Professor Walter Jackson Bates' course, "The Age of Johnson," had "the hardest exam I ever took at Harvard." I had decided to take the course anyway and have always been thankful that I did.

Today's Harvard students won't have the opportunity to browse through their own college course catalogs 40 or 50 years later, because the catalogs are now only available online. Even if they still have access to the electronic catalogs, they won't have handwritten notations in them.

18

The Mystery Plaque

My parents were visiting me at Harvard College on October 16, 1965, a day when I was scheduled to row in a major boat race. It was the first occurrence of Boston's now-famous "Head of the Charles" race. They stood on Anderson Bridge to watch my boat leave Newell Boathouse and head downriver.

When I returned from the race, my father showed me a small brass plaque on the bridge near where they were standing and asked if I knew what it was. I had never noticed it before, even though I had walked back and forth over that bridge twice every day while walking to and from rowing practice. It was easy to miss because it was near the sidewalk in an indented parapet. In addition, it was tarnished, was almost the size of the bricks, and had a few strands of ivy hanging over it.

The engraving on the plaque said:

Quentin Compson III
June 2, 1910
Drowned in the Fading of Honeysuckle

Although I had never seen the plaque before, I knew who Quentin Compson was. He was the fictional Harvard freshman in two of William Faulkner's novels, *The Sound and the Fury* and *Absalom, Absalom!* who died by suicide by jumping into the Charles River with flat irons tied to his feet.

There are rare masterworks of fiction that are so realistic or so moving that you wonder if the story they are telling is true. Seeing this plaque made me wonder if Quentin Compson's suicide, which already seemed realistic, had been based on a true event. It caused me go to look at archived issues of *The Harvard Crimson* from June 1910 to see if a suicide had been reported that month. I didn't find a report of a suicide, because the event was entirely fictional. It turns out that I was not the only person who felt that Quentin Compson's death seemed real. A *Washington Post* writer, Dale Russakoff, later wrote that Quentin Compson's "anguish is so personal and haunting that generations of readers have come to regard him as someone real."

Quentin Compson represented universal truths: the struggle of a young man with the ambiguities of the society he was born into, in this case in post-Civil War Mississippi; the struggle to accept that an earlier "Golden

Age" may never have really existed; and the struggle to reconcile good and beauty with coexisting evil. When Faulkner died in 1962, his obituary in *The Harvard Crimson* said: "Quentin . . . doubtless reflects some attributes of the archetypal Harvard student. ... But Quentin's dilemmas, Faulkner would insist, are not the dilemmas of the Harvard student, or even of the Southern student at Harvard. They are rather the 'old verities and truths of the heart.'"

In the weeks that followed, I made some inquiries about the plaque. None of my friends had seen it, nor had a few English instructors whom I asked. I took my English seminar group to see the plaque, and the instructor commented, "It's life imitating art." He was referring to the saying, "Life imitates art far more than art imitates life." His quip was certainly appropriate, if one considers that the plaque (life) was imitating the novels (art).

In the novels, Quentin Compson entered Harvard in the fall of 1909, in the Harvard College class of 1913. Many graduates in that class would later serve in World War I and some would die on the battlefields in Europe. But in this fictional world, time moved on without Quentin after his suicide in 1910, and the passage of time is one of Faulkner's themes here. Before Quentin left home to go to Harvard, his father gave him his grandfather's watch. Just before his suicide, he smashed the watch crystal (injuring himself) and removed the hands, but he noticed that the watch still went on ticking in his pocket though it would no longer tell him the time. He left a suicide note with the dismembered watch, smashed and bloody, in his Harvard room.

The plaque's inscription referred to "honeysuckle" because honeysuckle is a strong image in *The Sound and the Fury*; in some sections of the book, the word appears on almost every page. Faulkner mentions "a voice weeping steadily and softly beyond the twilit door the twilight-colored smell of honeysuckle," that "the air seemed to drizzle with honeysuckle;" in Boston, Quentin noted the absence of honeysuckle, thinking, "honeysuckle was the saddest odor of all."

Faulkner did not specify which bridge Quentin jumped off. Readers have assumed it was Anderson Bridge, which is the most prominent bridge at Harvard. It was built by Larz Anderson, a famous American diplomat, as a memorial to his father, Nicholas Longworth Anderson, a Civil War general. However, the construction of Anderson Bridge was not completed until 1915, so if Quentin Compson jumped off a bridge at Harvard it would most likely have been Great Bridge, which was located at that spot before Anderson Bridge.

For years after I noticed the plaque, it remained relatively unknown, and knowledge of it spread mainly by word-of-mouth. One American literature instructor, Kevin Starr, told his class about it in 1972 and mentioned that no one knew the plaque's origins. It was in Starr's class that the writer Russakoff learned about the plaque. Russakoff later described it as "a tarnished brass plaque . . . obviously was meant to be secret, so tiny and so obscured by vines and shadows that I had walked past it countless times without noticing."

The mystery remained: Who put the plaque there? Russakoff became the key to solving the mystery. Russakoff had told her mother, who lived in Birmingham, Alabama, about the mystery of the plaque. Her mother knew that their minister, Stanley Stefancic, had attended Harvard Divinity School and she told him about the plaque. To her surprise, Stefancic revealed that he himself had attached the plaque to the bridge using epoxy glue on June 2, 1965, the 55th anniversary of the suicide. He was helped by his wife, Jean, and his friend Tom Sugimoto, an MIT graduate student in physics. All three were non-Southerners who admired Faulkner's writing. They had hoped that an air of mystery would be associated with the plaque, and that only those who loved Faulkner's writing would discover the plaque and appreciate it. It appears that they succeeded.

An air of mystery continued to attach to the plaque. The plaque disappeared in 1983 during the 1978–1983 renovation of the bridge. Perhaps it disappeared into the waters of the Charles River, just as Quentin Compson had. The disappearance of the plaque was reported on television station WGBH on June 2, 1983, the 73rd anniversary of the suicide, and a few weeks later a replacement plaque appeared mysteriously and anonymously after dark, attached at the same spot where the original plaque had been.

However, the new plaque was made of cheaper metal and the wording had been changed to:

Quentin Compson
Drowned in the odour of honeysuckle
1891–1910

This change was highly controversial, and most observers objected to it. "Fading" had become "odour," often a more negative word, and it implied that Quentin was tormented by the smell of honeysuckle. Actually, Quentin *missed* the odor of honeysuckle, saying that the North had "the odor of summer and darkness except honeysuckle," which he missed, even though "honeysuckle was the saddest odor of all, I think." The poetry of the original inscription was gone; gone was the notion of a beautiful memory "fading," of something being lost, slowly and (because it was a suicide) irreversibly. It symbolized, in addition to the fading and loss of a memory, the fading and loss of youth. On the new plaque, the Roman numeral in Quentin's name was gone, making it less "real" somehow; and the dates of Quentin's life (1891–1910) had been added.

The mystery grew again; in 2014 the plaque again vanished during the 2012–2016 renovation of the bridge. Two years later, that second plaque was found (it had been found in the dirt in 2014 and then was forgotten for two years in a drawer). A new plaque (the third iteration, this time in brass) was created and attached by the Massachusetts Department of Transportation in 2017, with wording identical to the original plaque,

Quentin Compson III
June 2, 1910
Drowned in the Fading of Honeysuckle

Unlike the first two versions of the plaque, which had been mounted on the inside of the bridge wall, this third version was placed on the *outside* of the bridge. If you go to look for it, you can find it on the downstream side of the bridge, on the abutment at the Cambridge end of the bridge, ten rows of bricks above the granite base. Since this version was put there by the Massachusetts Department of Transportation, perhaps it will remain there indefinitely, for the fascination of readers of Faulkner for many years to come.

19

Long Before Pearl Harbor, an Entire Hospital Was Sent to Help England in World War II

Harvard University President James B. Conant had the idea of sending a fully staffed hospital to England to help the British in their war with Germany in 1939, more than two years before the US entered the war. It became a collaboration between Harvard University and the American Red Cross. They sent prefabricated hospital buildings, a team of Harvard doctors and laboratory technicians, a team of American Red Cross nurses, and laboratory and clinical equipment. The first physicians were sent in August, 1940.

The hospital was intended to provide medical care to infectious disease patients in southwest England and to investigate epidemics throughout the country. It was also intended to study how epidemics are transmitted between civilian and military populations in wartime.

Heavy bombing was expected, and large civilian crowds in air raid shelters for many hours might lead to epidemics, which could then spread to the military.

The entire project was dangerous. When the director of the hospital, Dr. John E. Gordon (previously Professor of Preventive Medicine and Epidemiology at Harvard Medical School) arrived in London, a falling bomb destroyed his apartment, and he suffered scalp injuries and bruises. As the days rolled on, Dr. Gordon noted the unearthly "day-in and day-out, night-in and night-out pounding, under which the British capital lives, the waiting for the banshee wail of the alarm . . . and the shattering of bombs, which one waits to fall."[1]

The Atlantic Crossing and Torpedoes

Everything for the new hospital had to be transported across the Atlantic in convoys guarded by warships. In regions of the Atlantic where submarine attacks were most likely, hospital staff were told to sleep in their clothes and to keep a life jacket and a small bag (with passport and first aid kit) nearby. They were asked to stay awake until 2 a.m. and take afternoon naps, so that they would be asleep for fewer of the dark hours when a submarine attack was more likely.[2]

In June 1941, a British convoy carrying 29 nurses for the hospital was attacked on its seventh day at sea. The SS *Vigrid*, which had been lagging due to engine trouble, was torpedoed and sunk. The 10 nurses on board were lowered into 3 lifeboats; one drifted for 12 days until rescued, one drifted for 19 days, and the third lifeboat, with 4 nurses, was never found. Eight days later, the SS *Maasdam* in another convoy was torpedoed and sunk; from that ship, the nurses' chaperone and one nurse were lost when their lifeboat sank.

Outside the American Red Cross headquarters at 17th and E Streets, NW, Washington, DC., you can see a plaque that says: "This plaque acknowledges the public spirit of Harvard University and the dedication of the staff of the American Red Cross–Harvard Field Hospital Unit." It lists the names of the American Red Cross nurses and their chaperone who died when their ships were torpedoed.

The Hospital

The hospital officially opened on September 22, 1941 on Salisbury Plain, 1½ miles from the city of Salisbury. Nearby there were large military training facilities including live firing ranges. The hospital consisted of 22 prefabricated buildings made of wood on steel frames, which had been shipped to England in 250,000 pieces in 30 ships. It had a capacity of 125 hospital beds.

The landscape in many parts of southwest England consists of chalk covered by a layer of turf. During construction, the exposed chalk on the ground made the location very visible to planes flying over, and "one had the uncomfortable feeling of living on a rather obvious target," in the words of one of the physicians.[3] Later, the chalk was covered again with topsoil, and fortunately, the hospital itself was never bombed.

There were three residential buildings with individual sleeping quarters for each staff member, as well as an administration building, a kitchen and dining room building, a recreation building, and a laboratory building. The recreation building had an assembly room, three parlors, a game room with ping pong, a kitchenette, and a library. There was also a "men's club room" for men only, about which one of the women wrote, "They need a retreat, poor dears, since the place will be overrun with women."[4]

The Staff

The American Red Cross-Harvard Field Hospital eventually had 10 physicians, 62 nurses, 6 technicians, and 8 administrative staff. Many of the physicians had been on the staff of Harvard Medical School or its hospitals, including two residents (one of whom, Paul Beeson, would later edit the two major internal medicine textbooks used by a generation of US physicians) and one clinical fellow.

Although the work was intense, there was also time off. The summer days were long because, from 1940 to

1945, England was on "double daylight savings time" in summer, i.e. two hours ahead of the peacetime clocks in winter. Letters[5] written to family back in the US describe bicycle rides after work to nearby villages and Roman ruins along the country lanes with high hedges on either side, surrounded by fields with wildflowers. On weekends they sometimes bicycled to Stonehenge, about 10 miles away. Dances, skits, and other gatherings were organized in the recreation room, and the staff sometimes went by bus to attend dances at other hospitals, or on weekends to London by train, about 80 miles away.

Medical and Scientific Contributions

In 1940, the infectious disease environment was very different from today. There were almost no antibiotics for civilian use, and there were fewer vaccines than today. The epidemiological staff of the hospital, known as the Harvard Public Health Unit, investigated infectious outbreaks throughout Great Britain and Northern Ireland, including outbreaks of scabies, trichinosis, paratyphoid fever, "epidemic respiratory disease," "epidemic myalgia," mumps, meningitis, typhoid fever, tuberculosis, and "food poisoning." They investigated an outbreak of smallpox in Glasgow. In early 1942, in parallel with similar investigations in the U.S., they investigated an outbreak of 1,591 cases of hepatitis among U.S. troops in Northern Ireland caused by a contaminated yellow fever vaccine. At least seven scientific papers about some of these investigations were published between 1941–1942 by the hospital staff.[6]

In 1941, the British Ministry of Health wrote to tell Harvard University management about one of these investigations:

> Let me tell you what happened in Bristol a few weeks ago. That city, which has suffered severely from air raids and whose health department has been seriously overworked, was visited by a widespread epidemic of paratyphoid fever. The resources of the city proved inadequate to the occasion, and Dr. Gordon was asked to help. He sent six of his nurses to the local isolation hospital to lend a hand there. Another six public health nurses, together with a doctor, took charge of the field work and two laboratory technicians undertook all the necessary laboratory work. As a result, the situation was brought rapidly under control, and Dr. Gordon earned the gratitude of the whole city.[7]

The hospital and its American doctors, nurses, and technicians also provided moral support for the British war effort. Dr. Gordon wrote in October, 1940: "The fact that Harvard University had made a formal and definite offer of medical assistance within a few weeks after the collapse of France – when British prospects appeared blackest – had created a profound impression . . . [and led to] excellent opportunities for service, both to a people who are bearing an unbelievable strain with marvelous fortitude, and in the advancement of medical knowledge."[8]

The US entered World War II in December 1941, and US forces were soon arriving in England to prepare for further battles. On July 15, 1942 the American Red Cross-Harvard Field Hospital was transferred to the US Army Medical Corps, and its laboratory became the central US military laboratory for the European theater of operations. At the time of the transfer, some of the hospital staff, including Dr. Gordon, joined the US Army; 30 of the nurses transferred to the U.S. Army Nurse Corps and 12 others continued to work in the UK as civilian nurses. After the war ended, the hospital buildings were given to the British government.

20

A Harvard Class in World War II

Even before the United States entered World War II in December 1941, war-related changes were in the air at colleges and universities throughout the US. The beginnings of World War II had been ongoing in China since July 1937 and in Europe since September 1939. Although some people in the US failed to notice the warning signs, many university administrators, including those at Harvard University, spent the tense months of 1940 and 1941 listening to war news and wanting to help the US prepare.

Harvard before Pearl Harbor

Harvard's president, James Conant, was one of those who was concerned. He contacted Vannevar Bush, head of the Carnegie Institution, to get him to give President Franklin Roosevelt his idea for creating a government science committee to give contracts to universities for science research for military preparedness. This led to formation of the National Defense Research Committee (NDRC), which Conant later chaired. Harvard began focusing on war-related research throughout its science facilities.[1] Beginning in 1939, Conant also organized sending an entire prefabricated hospital to England to assist them in the war, the first physicians arriving from Harvard Medical School in August 1940, and the hospital being fully functional by September 1941.[2]

Harvard alumni of the Class of 1937, attending their reunion in 1940,[3] recounted in their "Class Report" disturbing experiences while travelling during 1937–1940 that indicated they might have a war in their future. One classmate who travelled to Danzig, Poland, after war broke out there in 1939, spent five and a half days in a prison for having filmed German troops there. Another arrived in Shanghai on the first day of the war there and was "machine-gunned and bombed." Another visited Europe in 1937–1938 and wrote that "Europe on the eve of war had all the fascination of a dread, chromatic poison." One classmate wrote (in a later Class Report) that he joined the Navy before Pearl Harbor and survived the crippling explosion on the USS *Kearny* in its October 1941 battle with German U-boats in the North Atlantic, almost two months before US entry into the war. One classmate who had spent a year at Oxford on a Henry Fellowship was now "engaged in reading the war obituaries" of his former Oxford classmates.

Fifteen men from the Class of 1937 had already joined the armed services and thirteen had joined the reserves or National Guard by 1940. A few of these indicated they joined in order to have a more favorable situation when the war eventually came, which they clearly anticipated.

Changes on campus when war began

On Harvard's campus, most war-related changes began after Pearl Harbor. Many students were drafted, particularly after the draft age was lowered from 21 to 18 in November 1942; many faculty were drafted as well, and also many students and faculty volunteered for military service.

Harvard adopted a year-round academic calendar. Beginning in 1942, civilian freshmen could enter in either June or at the start of any semester, and they could graduate after two years and three months.[1]

In Harvard College there had been 1,400 civilian (male) freshmen in the fall of 1942; in the fall of 1943 there were only 500.[4] In part because of the smaller classes, Harvard began allowing women from Radcliffe College to enroll in upper level courses for the first time in 1943.[1] The daily student newspaper, *The Harvard Crimson*, was replaced by the semi-weekly *Harvard Service News*.[1] The student-run radio station offered some Morse code training.[1] Formal intercollegiate football was suspended from spring 1943 until the end of the war.[1]

Uniformed students marched in drills in Harvard Yard, inside Memorial Hall, and on the baseball diamond at Soldiers Field.[1] Sometimes, as "formations marched to class, martial music wafted over the Yard."[4]

Many campus facilities were turned over to the military (under contracts), including classrooms, laboratories, dormitories (Harvard Yard buildings, as well as Eliot, Kirkland, and Leverett Houses, and most of Winthrop House[1]), and dining halls. Harvard President Conant moved out of the official president's house on Quincy Street to allow its use for the headquarters of Navy training programs on campus. By the fall of 1942, more than 3,000 armed forces personnel were taking courses at Harvard,[5] military courses but also normal academic courses.[1]

Military courses that were added to the curriculum[1] included navigation, camouflage, meteorology, and the economic aspects of war. Military training programs in material procurement for supply officers, contracts (at the Harvard Business School), radar, and chaplaincy (in the Germanic Museum) were formed, as was a "School for Overseas Administration." Language courses were expanded. The Harvard School of Public Heath taught tropical medicine to Navy physicians.

Six members of the Class of 1937[6] were pleased to find that their Navy service began with a return to Harvard for two, three, or five months of training in the Navy "Electronics School," "Communications School," or "Supply Corps School." Three classmates who had graduated from the Harvard Business School (HBS), returned to HBS for the Supply Corps School. One arrived there one week after graduating from HBS, and another was "billeted in almost the same room in McCulloch Hall I had left two years earlier—but this time under Navy surveillance and strict Navy discipline."[6]

The changes brought by World War II to the Harvard campus have been described in articles and books, but the experiences of Harvard alumni fighting that war have not. These can be learned by an analysis of the experiences of one class, the Harvard Class of 1937, as told in their autobiographical essays in the 1947 "Class Reports."[6]

An example of Harvard alumni in combat: the Class of 1937

From the Class of 1937, 651 men out of 1,029 in the class (62%) served in the armed forces of the US or its Allies during World War II (Table I); 26 (4% of those on active duty) died in wartime service. They were among the more than 24,000 alumni[7] of Harvard College and Harvard graduate schools who served in the armed forces during World War II, of whom 697 (2.9%) died during the war.[1]

The members of the Class of 1937 had had time to reflect on their experiences by the time of their tenth reunion in 1947. For this reunion, in a tradition followed for all Harvard reunions, they wrote autobiographical essays that were published in a bound "Class Report." For

Table I. Approximate Distribution[a] of Armed Forces Enlistment of the Class of 1937 in World War II

Branch of Service	Number of Classmates	Percent of Those on Active Duty
Army[b]	374	57%
Navy	238	37%
Marine Corps	8	1%
Coast Guard	14	2%
US Public Health Service[c]	2	<1%
Armed forces of US Allies	9	1%
American Field Service[d]	2	<1%
Unspecified	6	1%
Total	**651**	

[a]The numbers in this table were compiled from multiple sources, including the autobiographical essays in the Class Report for 1947 and data from a questionnaire sent to classmates in 1947, and thus may be subject to minor inaccuracies. The total number on active duty, 651 classmates, is derived entirely from the autobiographical essays of 1947.

[b]Including sixty-four in the Army Air Force; there was no separate air force at that time.

[c]The US Public Health Service was "militarized" during World War II.

[d]Two classmates in the American Field Service were listed here as active duty because 1) these volunteer ambulance drivers were in uniform, 2) they served in the front lines, 3) one of them was killed by a mortar shell and was included in the list in the Class Report of those killed "for the cause of the Allies." A third classmate also was in the American Field Service until the fall of France in 1940 and later joined the Canadian army.

those who did not submit essays (including those who had died), biographies were written by others.

This Class Report opened with a somber two-page dedication to the twenty-six classmates who died "for the cause of the Allies in the Second World War," including a poem written by the mother of a classmate who died on active duty (Figure 1), which "expresses . . . our innermost feelings about friends and classmates who did not return from war."

Figure 1. Memorial Poem by the Mother of Walter Rosen, Class of 1937, Who Died on Active Duty, August 18, 1944

Farewell to a Flyer

Be still, dear restless heart, broke like thy wings, and
    breaking mine;
The genius from thy poor cracked skull is flown,
The deep eyes closed, that strained at knowledge
And saw worlds beyond the stars,
But see not me now: the long limbs still,
And all thy light gay grace, and mischievous smile,
Gone from this darker world, as when the sun
    has left.
    —Lucie Bigelow Rosen

Battles and Other Duty Assignments

The Class of 1937 fought in many of the war's major battles. Thirty-four classmates received eighty-two military awards for valor or meritorious service.

Two members of the class were in the US Navy at Pearl Harbor when the Japanese surprise attack occurred on December 7, 1941. One was on the USS *Tangier* and mentioned that his ship was the first to open fire on the Japanese planes; he was later an Attack Group Commander in the Allied invasion of Saipan.

In Asia, thirty-eight classmates fought in the Philippines. The actual number might be larger, since many others wrote that they had served "in the South Pacific." Six fought at Iwo Jima, including one who was the commanding officer of a tank landing ship (LST) in the initial assault, and nineteen fought at Okinawa. Some fought at Saipan and Tarawa; participated in the first carrier attack on the Inland Sea of Japan; served on multiple missions in B-29s over Japan; underwent kamikaze attacks (a classmate on one ship endured eighty-three air attacks in fifty-two hours, including kamikaze attacks); and one served in the Pacific on a submarine that sank two transports, two destroyers, and two freighters.

In Europe, one piloted a B-25 for fifty-four combat missions over Italy; another served as bombardier on forty-two combat missions. One shot down Luftwaffe torpedo bombers from a ship in the Mediterranean; others fought in the invasions of North Africa and Sicily, in the Ardennes (including two at the Battle of the Bulge) and at Remagen Bridge. One conducted advance landings behind enemy lines in preparation for the Anzio invasion; and one served with the "Special Allied Airborne Reconnaissance Force." Eleven classmates were part of the Normandy invasion and the battles to secure it.

Franklin Delano Roosevelt, Jr., one of President Roosevelt's sons, was in the Harvard Class of 1937. He served on destroyers in the Atlantic, Pacific, Caribbean, Mediterranean, and on the Murmansk run, and participated in the invasions of North Africa, Sicily, the Philippines, Iwo Jima, and Okinawa. He was executive officer of the destroyer USS *Mayrant*, and later was commander of the destroyer escort USS *U.M. Moore*. His essay modestly omits mention of his four awards for bravery that have been recounted elsewhere, including the Legion of Merit and a silver star for carrying a wounded sailor to safety under fire during the invasion of Sicily.

Fifty-five classmates worked in intelligence or counter-intelligence. Ten were assigned by the military to the Office of Strategic Services (OSS) and forty were in military intelligence and counter-intelligence services. One of these was an army psychiatrist working with OSS to select secret agents. Three civilian classmates also worked in OSS and two civilian classmates worked in other intelligence services.

Some classmates served on the staffs of prominent leaders, including the staffs of General George Marshall, Admiral Chester Nimitz, General Douglas MacArthur, Field Marshall Bernard Montgomery, and with Averell Harriman (US Ambassador to the Soviet Union) at the Teheran Conference. One classmate who was in the Free French Forces spent some time as General Charles De Gaulle's driver. Another was in the Military Police guarding President Roosevelt's home at Hyde Park.

As the war ended, some classmates were among the first US troops entering Tokyo, Yokohama, and Nagasaki, or were present in Tokyo Bay when Japan surrendered. When the fighting ended in Europe, one classmate was in charge of the military government of forty towns in Italy for two months in 1945.

Killed, Wounded, Sunk, or Captured

Twenty-six classmates died on active duty (4% of those on active duty). Thirteen (50%) of these died in plane crashes. Six died in land battles, two died in sea battles, one died of acute poliomyelitis and one died of scrub typhus. Twelve of the dead left behind a wife; seven also left behind one or more children.

One was killed by a sniper while leading his men through the woods in Germany. Another was killed while on a bombing mission over Yugoslavia. One classmate was in the Battle of Midway Island on the destroyer USS *Hammann*, which was sunk by a torpedo while fighting fires on the carrier USS *Yorktown*. He went into the water and was able to float clear of the sinking ship, but another explosion on the *Hammann* as it was going down killed him and other survivors in the water. Subsequently, a destroyer escort was named in his honor (USS *Lovering*) and served in the Pacific war.

Most of the war dead from the Class of 1937 were buried overseas. The entry for one classmate, who died in the crash of his fighter-reconnaissance aircraft and was buried in France, reported that "Father Maurice Colbert, the Parish priest, has reported to Wolf's father that his grave [in the Parish Cemetery at Cerisy-Belle-Etoile] is always well cared for and covered with flowers by the parishioners."

Nine other classmates were wounded in battle, including two seriously wounded during the Normandy invasion, and one who was wounded near Metz and required sixteen months of hospitalization. Five classmates were on ships that were sunk in battle, four of whom survived.

Three classmates were captured by the enemy. One was captured by the Germans in the Ardennes and was sent as a POW to Poland, later was marched to Bavaria when the Russians were approaching, and eventually was liberated by US troops; he required hospitalization for four months thereafter. One was captured by the Germans for nine hours in February 1945, possibly in Belgium, but then escaped, "unharmed, except for hurt dignity." One civilian classmate was a prisoner of the Japanese in Hong Kong for six months.

Civilian Classmates

There were 379 classmates (37%) who were not in the military during the war. Seven had died before 1940. Some others had medical deferments. Four were conscientious objectors who performed alternative public service in national forests, state mental institutions, and elsewhere. One other was initially a conscientious objector but later "finally decided I was no longer a pacifist at all," joined the army, and was assigned to OSS. Eighty-three were doing work that might have exempted them from military service, including four FBI agents (one of whom did intelligence work in France and Germany), three in OSS, two in other intelligence services, five in the US foreign service, twenty-two in various military or government offices, seventeen working or supervising in factories making aircraft, tanks, or other military hardware, two in the merchant marine, and eighteen in war-related research on radar, chemical warfare, burns, or malaria.

Discussion

From the Harvard College Class of 1937, 651 men served in the armed forces in World War II (62% of the entering class of 1,029), and twenty-six died on active duty (4% of those on active duty). The classmates described these experiences in essays for the 1947 Class Report that were written while the memories were still fresh. Their wartime contributions also can be considered as representative of the war service of alumni from other Harvard classes, and probably also of alumni of other universities. Their service was important for the success of the US war effort.

21

Things I Noticed on
the Day Robert Kennedy Was Buried

On June 8, 1968, I was among a small group of students who had been asked to be ushers at the burial of Senator Robert F. Kennedy at Arlington National Cemetery a few days after his assassination. His funeral had been held that morning in New York City, and his casket was being taken by train to Washington, D.C.

We were told to arrive at Arlington before sunrise although the casket was not expected until 4:30 p.m. When I arrived, Secret Service agents with visible shoulder-holsters under their suit jackets were already standing near the freshly dug grave in the pre-dawn dimness. I was given a fold-back lapel pin to identify me as someone allowed into the area.

Customs agents and park police in plain clothes arrived after sunrise to supplement the Secret Service. The agents from the three services all knew each other by first names, and they told me they had worked together before. The customs agents looked like intimidating waterfront characters but they were particularly friendly.

The bright early morning light shone on the open gravesite that was located in the middle of three concentric rope cordons. Suddenly, a strange man appeared between the outermost cordons; no one had noticed how he arrived—he seemed to arise from the ground itself. He was tall, with slick hair, wearing a dark suit, a shirt with a Nehru collar, and had a satanic appearance. He carried a black brief case. The Secret Service agents ordered him to open the briefcase, which contained only an advanced camera. To my surprise, they sent him away without questioning him, and laughed about him afterwards.

The cemetery remained empty most of the day. However, the singer Bobby Darin arrived with a bodyguard around 11 a.m. and sat throughout the day under a large oak tree, apparently grieving. He had become concerned with society's problems in recent months and must have had some contact with Robert Kennedy. Everyone recognized him, but by whispered agreement they allowed him to sit privately. At noon, an army jeep drove one of the students to a local MacDonald's to bring back lunch for everyone, though Darin and his bodyguard left separately to get their own lunch and returned to the oak tree.

The day became very hot. During the afternoon, some rain fell. We took shelter under the porch of a building on the cemetery grounds until the sun returned.

The burial was supposed to occur at the end of the afternoon, and large numbers of people started to arrive as the time approached. However, the train bringing the casket was delayed because of enormous crowds of mourners all along the train's route. Late in the afternoon there was a further delay when a man and a woman who were waiting along the route were killed by another train on the adjacent tracks. A child the woman was carrying was thrown clear and lived. I wondered how the story of this day would be told to the child when he or she grew up.

An enormous floral arrangement on a tripod was placed about 50 feet from the gravesite; it was a solid circle of flowers with a floral number "7" in it. Someone said this was a funeral ritual for members of "The Seven Society," a secret society at the University of Virginia Law School, where Kennedy had been a student.

The funeral train reached Union Station after 9 p.m. A procession of cars with the casket crossed the river to Arlington Cemetery and drove up the winding road on the cemetery hillside. As the casket arrived, dignitaries arrived separately: President Johnson, Vice-President Humphrey, senators, congressmen, and cabinet officers stepped out of limousines onto the walkway. Everyone remained standing in the dark during the brief service, lit only by a full moon, a few lights, and the photographers' flashbulbs, with plain-clothes agents around them and uniformed police on the roadside nearby. I was struck by the concentration of power and responsibility in this small space, and its vulnerability, protected only by a human shield with handguns. So many of the U.S. leaders were together on this exposed knoll, and although it was a military cemetery, there were no soldiers in evidence. In retrospect, I am now also surprised that both the President and Vice President were in one public place at the same time, and that President Johnson was there at all, given his known animosity toward Robert Kennedy.

The graveside service began around 10:30 p.m. This was the first burial to be held at night at Arlington Cemetery in anyone's memory. The service was brief, with few words and no rifle volley. The dignitaries returned in the dark to their limousines, and the limousines left.

As the dignitaries left, I ran into Mary-Jo Kopechne, one of Robert Kennedy's secretaries, on the walkway, with whom I had worked in Robert Kennedy's office in previous summers. She looked stricken, and barely responded when I said something. The next year she would be killed in a car driven by Robert Kennedy's other brother, Senator Edward Kennedy, when it drove off a small bridge at Chappaquiddick Island.

Someone gave me a ride down to the parking lot where I had left my own car about 16 hours earlier. As we slowly drove down the winding cemetery drive, I suddenly noticed hundreds of small lights flickering on the hillside beyond the cordon. It took me a few seconds to realize that these were candles held by hundreds of people standing in the dark, mourning silently.

22

The Obituary Reader

I began reading newspapers before I entered junior high school. A few years later, an adult I knew, hearing that I liked to read newspapers, asked me what parts I liked. When I told him I liked the obituaries, he asked, "Aren't you too young to be reading obituaries?"

I understood what he meant, because even at that time, I realized that many adults read obituaries to find out which of their acquaintances have died. Later, I also realized that some people read obituaries with a feeling of "at least it's not me." The poet Donald Hall[1] once wrote that prior to age 70, he always looked at the age in the obituary and felt relief if he himself was younger. At some point in his seventies, he said, he stopped checking the age.

A good newspaper obituary always tells a good story. Here are a few examples of obituaries whose biographical stories could compete with any good short story.[2]

One obituary described a woman who had had four husbands. The first one, she said, was her "practice husband;" the second was "not a great husband, but gave me the best children;" the third was the love of her life; and the fourth, whom she married when she was 79, was "the perfect husband for that time of my life." She freely dispensed similar wisdom to others. She advised a young woman about a pending marriage, "I've talked to [your fiancé] for a bit and can assure you that he'd make a fine first husband." Another young friend of hers was quoted as saying, "She gave me a foolproof method to get asked to dance. She said, you simply go up to the boy you want, wag your finger and say, 'Ooh, what I heard about you!' It worked like a charm. Only as we danced, the boy kept asking me what it was I had heard." And she didn't have an answer.

An obituary of a man who called himself "Poppa Neutrino," described his travels around the US in "a state of exuberant homelessness" with his children, performing together as a "busking street band." They usually lived on rafts made of old timbers and discarded plastic. In 1998, he crossed the Atlantic in a 60-day voyage on a 51-foot raft made from trash, accompanied by his fourth wife, three crew members, and three dogs. (His "exuberant homelessness" must have contributed to his having had four wives.) The raft survived storms and near-collisions with ships and icebergs. It was his second successful raft trip across the Atlantic, but it was the first time on a raft made of trash. The philosophy driving him, he said, was that "I had an intuitive knowledge that human life was 99 percent defeat, and that you had to do something extraordinary to turn it into victory."

An obituary of an American fighter pilot in World War II said he was known as "King of the Strafers" because he had shot down 15 enemy aircraft. He himself was ultimately shot down over Germany and was threatened with execution, but was offered a drink before being shot. He spotted a box of Havana cigars, asked for one of those instead of the drink, and surprised the soldier who had captured him by blowing smoke rings. His captor had never seen anything like this and so he taught his captor to blow smoke rings. In the end he was sent to a prison camp instead of being shot. He later commented, "People say smoking costs lives. It saved my life."

One obituary was for a man who had been a piano prodigy and had broadcast from Radio City Music Hall at age 5. However, he had always wanted to be a spy and eventually applied for a job at the Central Intelligence Agency (CIA). However, he went to the wrong address for his CIA interview and never became a spy.

A woman who had never thought about being a reporter became a fearsome investigative reporter. While she was still a housewife, the editor of a newspaper in Florida asked if she would like to be their correspondent in a nearby town. She replied, "I've never written anything. Why would you come to me?" The editor said that the local librarian told him that she checked out more books than anybody else. He assumed that if she liked literature, she would be able to write the news. She went on to become a successful investigative reporter, bringing down corrupt police, bringing down a drug ring, and enhancing protections for journalists who refuse to disclose anonymous sources. She would invite politicians to her house for a home-cooked meal to get tips on corruption. She once got tips slipped to her under the door of a department store dressing room.

Sometimes the best part of an obituary is the final sentence or two, usually a quotation. Some examples are:

- A Japanese nationalist politician said he liked governing and did not want to retire, "because I want to do what I like for the rest of my life, even if people hate me when I die."

- A Secret Service agent assigned to guard Henry Kissinger was asked by Kissinger, "What would you do if we were attacked by terrorists trying to kidnap me?" The agent responded, "I have my instructions, sir. You are not to be taken alive."

- A medical researcher received news of an improvement in his own health, and said, "I got a grant renewal!"

- A music promoter said, "I didn't ask for my life. It just happened. Very fortunate, I guess."

Someone once said that anyone who is over 100 years old will probably live forever, because you rarely see any obituaries for people older than 100. However, reading obituaries makes one think about how long one would actually wish to live. Someone asked the poet Donald Hall how long he would like to live, and he casually replied, "Oh, until eighty-three." After that he was very anxious until his eighty-fourth birthday had passed. (He lived to be 89.)

Donald Hall also commented that "If a person lives into old age, there's a moment when he or she becomes eldest in the family, perched on top of a hill as night rises."

23

Obituaries of Spies

In the leading East Coast newspapers,[1] there are often obituaries of former officials of the Central Intelligence Agency (CIA) and its predecessor, the Office of Strategic Services (OSS). This might be due only to the interests of the obituary writers or perhaps it reflects the ease of getting CIA stories from grieving relatives who are now relieved not to have to keep them secret any longer. We will not see many OSS obituaries in the future, because anyone who was old enough to have been in the OSS when it was operating (1942–1945) would be at least 96 years old at the time of this writing (2023). The OSS obituaries have a special historical flavor.

One young woman working at OSS, who had grown up in a mountaintop villa near Bologna, Italy, reviewed a message from partisans stating that the villa was being used by Nazi troops as a headquarters and observation point, and that the owners, her Italian relatives, had been restricted to a small part of the property. The message came with a request that it be bombed. She said later, "I couldn't notify my uncle and aunts and cousins. I could only pray!" In the end, the bombs missed their target and her relatives survived the war.

In another obituary, the deceased had been an OSS agent who was in a 1945 parachute commando mission to liberate a Japanese POW camp in Manchuria, China. One of the prisoners was his own father, who had been a prisoner there for three years. When the commandos arrived, his father said, "Son, what took you so long?"

Gold coins were a vital part of OSS operations, especially behind enemy lines. One OSS pilot flew night flights over Italy in a plane painted black, dropping supplies for undercover operatives behind enemy lines, including 500-pound containers full of gold coins. Years later, another agent, a CIA employee, was sent to recover hundreds of these "bail-out kits" containing gold coins that had been buried across Germany during World War II.

In some cases, the work for the OSS or the CIA was mundane, but those agents also clearly felt that the work was a highlight of their lives. One obituary described a CIA employee's work translating intercepted phone conversations of Joseph Stalin. One Associated Press writer working for the CIA from 1957 to 1980 said that his work was to provide official-looking press credentials as cover for CIA agents. Another CIA official arranged secret funding of the AFL-CIO, the National Student Association, and a European tour for the

Boston Symphony Orchestra as a way of supporting anti-communist activity. An obituary of a US geneticist who worked in Chongqing, China in 1943 reported that while there, he met Ilya Tolstoy, the grandson of Leo Tolstoy, who was working there for the OSS.

One agent, Peter Matthiessen, who was the author of more than 30 books and a writer for the *New Yorker*, founded a new literary magazine, *The Paris Review*, as cover for himself as a CIA agent in Paris. The magazine had staying power, became very popular in the literary world, and it remains so today.

"Special operations" are sometimes a feature of espionage. One obituary described a CIA station chief in the Congo who was trying to get control of Congo's cobalt, which was needed for missiles. He received a packet of poisons, including poisoned toothpaste, to be used to assassinate Patrice Lumumba, Congo's prime minister. Instead of following orders, he hid the poisons in his office safe (with a note of warning attached in case anyone got into his safe). Another former CIA officer helped train 300 Tibetan nationalists in guerilla warfare in the Colorado mountains and sent them by parachute into Tibet to fight against the Chinese occupation. He later became the "CIA officer in residence at the John F. Kennedy School of Government at Harvard University;" one can only wonder what his duties were in that post. Another former CIA employee, who later was one of the Watergate burglars (Bernard Barker), was quoted as saying that when he was applying to work for the CIA, he had to demonstrate his nerve and skills by breaking into the offices of Radio City Music Hall in New York without being detected.

An obituary for one CIA agent claimed he was the only CIA officer to recruit and run agents in both Beijing and Moscow. He spoke fluent Chinese and Russian, and liked to recite Chinese poetry. He made it a requirement that all operations officers make a parachute jump at 1,200 feet, but he also put great emphasis on meeting with agents on the ground in the streets of Moscow and Beijing. When he retired from the CIA, he received a retirement gift from his Russian adversaries: a coffee-table book printed by the Russians consisting entirely of surveillance photos they had taken of him driving or walking down the streets of Moscow.

The experiences of Bernard Knox as a US Army captain assigned to OSS operating behind enemy lines in Italy changed the course of his life. In a bombed-out farmhouse he noticed a gilt-edged copy of the works of the ancient Roman poet Virgil. He picked it up and remembered enough school Latin to sit there reading Virgil's description of war written 2,000 years earlier. The wisdom in it seemed so relevant to his current war situation, that he vowed that if he survived the war, he would study the classics. After the war, he earned a PhD in classics and became a professor and noted scholar of the classics at Yale.

Like everyone else, former spies eventually die and some of them appear in obituaries. Sometimes the obituaries include information that is no longer secret, adding fascinating footnotes to history.

24

African Slaves in the North

We were taught in school that there were few African slaves in the northern US colonies because slavery would only "work" in the South, where plantations and the hot weather made it practical. However, there were in fact many African slaves in the northern colonies throughout the 1600s and 1700s. There had been a shortage of labor there that could not be met by immigrant free laborers and indentured servants, so the northern colonial governments permitted the use of African slaves to fill the gap. In addition, an increase in deaths of White men during Queen Anne's War against the French and Indians (1702–1713) and during a smallpox outbreak (1721) worsened the labor shortage. In 1740, one in five families in Boston owned African slaves and African slaves represented 10% of the city's population. In 1790, African slaves made up more than 6% of the population in New York State (7.1% in New York City) according to the US Census in that year.

Slavery in New England began in 1637. In that year, the Pequod Indians attacked the colonists in Connecticut, and a force was sent to suppress them. The Indian women and children who were not killed were enslaved in New England. The Indian men who were not killed were considered too dangerous to keep in New England, so they were exchanged in the West Indies for African slaves who were brought back to New England, as recorded in 1638 in the journal of John Winthrop, the governor of Massachusetts. This was fully established as a policy in 1646, when the New England Confederation, a military alliance of several New England colonies, decided that hostile Indians could "be shipped out and exchanged for Negroes."

Soon the "Triangle Trade" developed, a cyclical trading arrangement in which merchants in the northern colonies bought sugar and molasses in the West Indies, used that to make rum in New England, and traded the rum, iron, and various other manufactured goods for slaves in Africa, sold the slaves in the West Indies, and then with the proceeds bought sugar and molasses to start the cycle again. Some of the slaves were also brought to New England. The powerful New England distilling and shipping industries that developed from this arrangement had a strong interest in maintaining the slave trade, and the slave trade helped build numerous family fortunes in New England.

Boston was the primary port for the slave trade in the United States during the 1600s, but other northern cities also became active slave ports in the 1700s. These cities were the focus of buying slaves and selling them to slave markets, from which they were ultimately sold to plantations in the southern colonies. When slaves were sold for local use in the North, they were not usually sold in slave markets, but were sold directly from the ships they arrived in. Newspaper advertisements for slaves appeared in 50–75% of issues of the major Boston newspapers during the 1700s, advertising the sale of slaves in Boston from ships they arrived in. In addition, many slaves were sold from private homes where they lived with their owners. Some were sold in taverns. Some advertisements directed potential buyers to contact the seller through the post office or through the printer of the newspaper.

A French traveler in 1688 wrote that "there is not a house in Boston, however small may be its means, that has not one or two [African slaves]," although the total number of slaves in Boston at the time suggests he was referring only to the houses of wealthy citizens. One historian has written that "the register of New England's aristocracy would serve as a roll call of Puritan slave owners," and a list of the 162 families with the most slaves in New England in the 1600s and 1700s includes the most recognizable historical New England family names. In 1706, Cotton Mather, the noted Boston clergyman and a leader in the community, recorded in his diary that members of his church bought him an African slave as a gift. Benjamin Wadsworth, president of Harvard College from 1729–1737, owned slaves. Almost 300 years later in 2016, Harvard University placed a plaque in remembrance of four African slaves who served Wadsworth and his successor, Edward Holyoke, president of Harvard College from 1737–1769. At the same time, some prominent Bostonians such as John Adams and Samuel Adams refused to own slaves.

African slaves in Boston played a key role in the introduction of variolation, an early form of smallpox prevention, several years before the famous introduction of variolation to Britain from Constantinople by Lady Mary Wortley Montagu. One slave was the source of the inoculation concept and two other slaves were experimental subjects of the first "clinical trial" of it in Boston. Sometime between 1706–1716, Cotton Mather's African slave Onesimus told him that in Africa old smallpox scabs were inoculated into people who had not yet had smallpox, to give a mild infection and confer future protection against smallpox. Mather convinced Dr. Zabadiel Boylston to try this in Boston during the smallpox epidemic of 1721, and Boylston performed the first inoculations in Boston on his six-year-old son and two of his slaves. (Thus, it is evident that both Mather and Boylston owned slaves in Boston.)

Pennsylvania's large Quaker community included some of the earliest opponents of slavery in the colonies, but slaves were present in Pennsylvania at least until the early 1800s even though a state law outlawed slavery there in 1790. The Civil War diarist Mary Chestnut wrote in 1861 that her mother-in-law from Philadelphia said to her, "Did you not know that my father owned slaves in Philadelphia? In his will he left me several of them." Mary Chestnut then commented in her diary, "In the Quaker city, and in the lifetime of a living woman now present, there were slaveholders. It is hard to believe." She adds with irony, "Time works its wonders of change like enchantment. So quickly we forget."

In New York, slaves were still present at least through the early 1800s. Doris Kearns Goodwin, in her book *A Team of Rivals*, describes how William Henry Seward, Lincoln's anti-slavery Secretary of State, born in 1801, grew up among his family's slaves in Orange County, New York. His New York neighbors also owned slaves; Seward recalled that a slave child owned by a neighbor was whipped, ran away, and was brought back in an iron yoke around his neck, before subsequently escaping permanently. Sojourner Truth, the African American abolitionist and feminist, was born into slavery in New York State, around 1797; she was sold multiple times within New York before she was freed by the New York law that outlawed slavery in 1827.

As time passed, more and more slaves in the northern states were freed by their owners. In the late 1700s, many citizens in the North found slavery to be incompatible with the ideals of the American Revolution

(1776–1783). There were economic pressures as well. During the 1700s, complex economic factors drove down the price of slaves in the northern colonies, so that it became more profitable to sell the slaves in the West Indies than to sell them in the northern colonies. By 1790, the US Census reported that 78% of Africans living in New England (13,059 of 16,822) were free and 22% (3,763) were slaves. By that year, slavery had diminished but persisted in New England.

African slaves were a part of life in the southern parts of the United States until the end of the Civil War, but they were also a part of life in the northern colonies throughout the 1600s and 1700s, and to a lesser extent in the years between the American Revolution and the Civil War. The buying and selling of slaves had deep roots in New England and was tightly integrated into the shipping and distillery industries and the overall economy there. In the North, as in the South, many White Americans would have seen African slaves during the course of their daily lives in colonial times and in the early years of the United States.

25

Two Great
European Writers Who
Were Descendants of African Slaves

Two famous European writers were descendants of African slaves. Alexandre Dumas' father was born into slavery in what is now Haiti. Alexander Pushkin's great-grandfather was born in Africa, enslaved as a child, taken to Constantinople, and then taken to Russia.

Dumas' father rose from slavery to become one of Napoleon's most successful generals, and Pushkin's great-grandfather rose from slavery to become a general in the Russian army. Thus, both rose in European society by excelling in the military and this made it easier for their descendants, the writers Dumas and Pushkin, to achieve social and literary success. Nevertheless, although their social status and the enlightened atmosphere of both Paris and St. Petersburg in the nineteenth century allowed each writer to flourish, there is evidence that each of them found it awkward to be a Black man in nineteenth-century Europe.

Alexandre Dumas

Alexandre Dumas ("Alexandre Dumas, père," 1802–1870) was the author of novels that are still widely read, including *The Three Musketeers, The Count of Monte Cristo,* and *The Man in the Iron Mask.* His grandfather was a White French aristocrat who went to what is now Haiti, where he fathered four children with a woman of African descent whom he purchased and lived with. He later returned to France with his 14-year-old son from that relationship, Thomas-Alexandre. Thomas-Alexandre later enlisted in the French army, rose to become one of Napoleon's most successful generals, and was key to Napoleon's victories in Italy. He personally led a commando raid that breached the enemy defenses in northern Italy. Eventually, he became so close to Napoleon that they discussed military matters together while Napoleon was in bed with his wife Josephine. However, Thomas-Alexandre later had a falling out with Napoleon. When Thomas-Alexandre died, Napoleon blocked the pension for his widow, so his son, the writer Alexandre Dumas, grew up in poverty.

At age 14, Alexandre Dumas left school to go to Paris to work as a scribe. He had a secret reason for moving to Paris: he wanted to write plays like the ones he had seen given by travelling companies in the countryside, and he quickly succeeded. Despite starting in poverty, by age 25 he had become one of the most popular playwrights in France. He was so popular that on at least one occasion his coat was ripped to shreds by an enthusiastic audience.

He also participated in two anti-royalist revolutions in Paris, one when he was 28 years old (in 1830) and one when he was 30 (in 1832), but he was not in any battles. After the revolution of 1832, he was warned that he was in danger of arrest, so he quickly left for Switzerland. For the next seven years, he worked as a very popular travel writer.

He began writing historical novels in 1838, at age 36. He eventually wrote 347 novels, a number so large that it invited accusations that he had not written them himself. He did, however, work with the help of a historian who provided historical background material for his novels.

Nevertheless, it is well-documented that he wrote during most of his waking hours. He wrote constantly, slept little, and ate quickly. He had lunch brought in on a trolley so he could eat without having to stop writing. When he went out in the evening to see a play or for dinner, he wrote again when he returned home. A cartoonist at the time drew a picture of Dumas writing at his desk with four separate pens between the fingers of each hand while a servant ladled soup into his mouth.

He described himself as a novelist working in a historical framework. "I start by devising a story . . . I search through the annals of the past to find a frame in which to set it; and it has never happened that history has failed to provide this frame, so exactly adjusted to the subject that it seemed it was not a case of the frame being made for the picture, but that the picture had been made to fit into the frame."

He became very wealthy, built a large country house where he gave lavish parties, and frequently gave money to friends and strangers, although he eventually lost most of his wealth. He was respected and loved in France, but he was also very conscious of being a Black man.

Dumas was reluctant to visit the United States, where he knew that he would not be treated well because of being Black. In 1864, the US consul in Paris asked Dumas to give a lecture tour in the US, despite the ongoing Civil War where a major issue was Black slavery. The consul reported to the State Department that Dumas "has been in doubt . . . whether we had sufficiently conquered our negrophobia to receive a person of mixed blood as [respectfully as] he is accustomed to be received in France."

However, Dumas also clearly saw the ambiguity of his position as a Black man even in France. At one time, he advised a young Black servant of his who was leaving to join the army, "Be a good soldier, rise to be a field-marshal and then, black as you are, everyone will swear you are white."

Alexander Pushkin

Alexander Pushkin (1799–1837) is considered by Russians to be their greatest poet. He is best known in the English-speaking world for his verse novel *Eugene Onegin*, for his play *Boris Gudonov*, and for a gripping short story, "The Queen of Spades."

Pushkin's great-grandfather was born in Africa and was sold as a slave in Constantinople at age five. A Russian official bought him and his brother as gifts for the Russian Czar Peter the Great. Czar Peter named him "Abram," arranged for his baptism (with Peter himself as godfather), and arranged for his education, which included military training in France. Abram then rose through the Russian army under Peter's successors, to become "General Abram Petrovich Gannibal, cavalier of the orders of St. Anne and Alexander Nevsky." He was in charge of all military engineering in Russia, and owned a large estate.

The writer Pushkin was born three generations later, and the family was still prominent in Russian society. (In addition to Pushkin's mother being a descendant of Peter the Great's godson Abram, his father was a member of the minor Russian nobility.) The family's several estates produced agricultural products that supported their aristocratic lifestyle. Pushkin attended a palace boarding school created by Czar Alexander I to train Russia's future leaders.

After graduation, Pushkin worked in the Foreign Ministry in St. Petersburg, and led a dissolute life, with gambling, many romances, and many duels. He wrote plays, short stories, romantic poems and poems about liberty, but he also wrote poems that mocked the czar. Eventually Czar Alexander decided he had tolerated Pushkin's behavior long enough, and exiled him from St. Petersburg. Pushkin spent the next six years (1820 to 1826) in internal exile, living successively in the Caucasus, in the Crimea, and on his family estates south of St. Petersburg. He was fortunate in not being exiled to Siberia, and perhaps this leniency resulted from being an aristocrat and already a famous poet.

A few years later, Pushkin's friendships with revolutionaries nearly got him into much more serious trouble. He was friends with at least ten members of the Decembrists, who attempted to overthrow the Czar in 1825; these friends included the five leaders who were hanged and two others who were sentenced to long prison terms. The only reason Pushkin had not also been involved in the plot was because his friends felt he could not be trusted to keep secrets.

But Pushkin's poetry had influenced the leaders of the plot. One of the hanged leaders said during an interrogation, "I heard everywhere Pushkin's verse being read with enthusiasm. This more and more strengthened my liberal opinions." Another leader wrote, "Who among the youth with anything of an education has not read and been carried away by the works of Pushkin, which breathe freedom!" The government conducted an investigation of Pushkin's loyalty in 1826, but in the end they found no reason to arrest him.

When Czar Alexander died in 1826, his successor, Czar Nicholas I, ended Pushkin's exile. Pushkin returned to St. Petersburg and five years later, at age 32, married a beautiful 19-year-old woman from Moscow. She was admired by the czar and by everyone at the court. Later, a Guards officer tried to seduce her, the seduction failed, but Pushkin fought a pistol duel with the Guards officer in which Pushkin was killed at age 37.

Pushkin had had a privileged position in Russian society, as well as literary success and romantic success with Russian women. He was liked by most people who knew him, including most other Russian writers. Nevertheless, he was clearly aware of his awkward position as a Black man in Russia at that time – even though he was an aristocrat. His friends and acquaintances clearly liked and admired him, but some of their surviving letters and diaries are racially disparaging, and Pushkin must have sensed these feelings. These documents demonstrate that nineteenth-century Russia was not a color-blind society. Pushkin lived his entire life as a free man in Russia, from 1799 to 1837. However, if he had lived in the United States in the same years, he most likely would have been a slave.

Nineteenth-century Russia did not have slaves, but it had a system of serfdom with many similarities to the slave system in the United States. Although serfs were not racially distinct from other Russians, they were bought and sold with the land, could be mortgaged, could be hired out by their owners, could be used by an owner to fulfill conscription quotas for the army, and were subject to sexual exploitation. Pushkin himself owned hundreds of serfs, mortgaged most of them, and fathered a child with the teenage daughter of one of his serfs.

Conclusions

These two great European writers, Dumas and Pushkin, had recent ancestors who were African slaves. Their literary success occurred because the societies in Paris and St. Petersburg allowed them to flourish. Their paths were made easier by the elite status of their families, which was due in large part to the military successes of their emancipated forefathers. Most western societies have a high regard for military success; the fact that their forefathers became generals contributed to the societies ignoring some misgivings related to race. Nevertheless, both Dumas and Pushkin were conscious that these societies were not color-blind.

26

Time and Punishment

Time appears to be linear and to be moving in one direction, but is it really? And punishment, in our culture, is usually linear: when it is given, it is almost always given after, not before, an offense. Similarly, rewards are usually given after a good deed or a kindness, not before. The linear nature of punishment and reward, as viewed in most cultures, depend on there being linearity of time.

At first glance, it is easy to think of time being linear because it appears to go in one direction. Most events seem to occur one after the other unless they are simultaneous. We see ourselves as being located at the "now" time point, somewhere between the known "past" behind us and the unknown "future" that we are facing. This linearity of time is part of our spoken and written culture. We talk about "timelines." We say that we "look back" at the past and "look forward" to the future. We remember the past, but not the future. It is also noteworthy that we have never observed time to reverse direction.

We sometimes speak of time as a flowing river, using a metaphor that has been in use since antiquity. The ancient Greek philosopher Heraclitus (who lived around 500 BC) saw time as being like a river, and said that "you cannot go into the same water twice."[1] Nowadays, it is common for this to be quoted as, "No man ever steps into the same river twice, for it's not the same river and he's not the same man." The Roman philosopher-emperor Marcus Aurelius (121–180 AD), who was an admirer of the works of Heraclitus, wrote, "Time is a river, the resistless flow of all created things. One thing no sooner comes in sight than it is hurried past and another is borne along, only to be swept away in its turn."[2] Some more recent writers have also seen time as a river, for instance Homer Smith in his book *Kamongo* (1932) and Thomas Wolfe in *Of Time and the River* (1935).

However, there have been alternative ways of looking at time. For instance, an analysis of ancient Greek writings by the Yale classics scholar Bernard Knox[3] showed that at least some of the ancient Greek writers thought of the past and present as being in front of them, because they could see and know the events that had occurred in the past or were occurring in the present. According to Knox, they thought of the future as being behind them because they could not see the events it held. They still thought of time as being linear and flowing in one direction, but they saw the position of the observer as standing in the present and facing the past.

Yet another view is that we are moving linearly within a framework of time, like moving along a road on a map. In this view, the past, present, and future exist simultaneously in various places on the map and are always present. All things on this map might exist simultaneously, and the past never disappears completely. The most mystical part of the Bible, the *Book of Revelation*,[4] says, "I am the Alpha and Omega, the beginning and the ending, . . . which is, and which was, and which is to come . . . "

Albert Einstein saw support for this concept in the laws of physics. He wrote in a letter about a friend who had died, who "has departed from this strange world a little ahead of me. That means nothing. For us believing physicists, the distinction between past, present, and future is only a stubborn illusion."[5]

We usually view both punishment and reward as linear, following the pattern of time. If punishment or reward are given at all, they usually follow an event that they are given for. However, if one takes the view that time is like a road on a map on which past, present, and future exist simultaneously, then punishment or reward theoretically could be given *before* the event that elicits it, as easily as after. This could also make it reasonable for forgiveness to precede a transgression.

References,
Notes, and Sources

References, Notes, and Sources

Medicine and Science

2. A Hispanic Amulet Against Disease in Infants

1. Irving W. "Legend of the Two Discreet Statues," in *Tales of The Alhambra*. Granada: Miguel Sanchez, 1973, pages 267–284.

2. Jones BJ. *Washington Irving: An American Original*. New York: Arcade Publishing, 2008, pages 251, 260.

3. Irving W. *Tales of the Alhambra*. Granada: Miguel Sanchez, 1973.

3. Learning the Vocabulary of Medicine (and Other Foreign Languages)

1. Morrison DA. *Different Drummer*. Altona, MB, Canada: Friesen Press, 2021. Pages 53, 79.

2. Sobel RK. "MSL – Medicine as a second language." *N Engl J Med* 2005; 352:1945–1946.

3. Hall FH. *Memories Grave and Gay*. New York: Harper, 1918, page 78.

4. Winterbotham FW. *The Nazi Connection*. New York: Dell, 1978, pages 169–170.

5. Macintyre B. *The Spy and the Traitor*. New York: Crown, 2018, page 102.

6. McLaughlin ME. "One hundred pages of music, no problem." *The Washington Post*, January 9, 2008.

7. Kidder T. *Mountains Beyond Mountains*. New York: Random House, 2009, page 113.

8. "List of anatomy mnemonics." Wikipedia 2023. Viewed at https://en.wikipedia.org/wiki/List_of_anatomy_mnemonics.

9. Hagerty JR. "Professor studied how elite performers reach the top." Obituary of Anders Ericsson. *Wall Street Journal*, June 27–28, 2020.

10. Foer, J. "Forget me not: How to win the U.S. memory championship." *Slate*, posted March 16, 2005; viewed at http://.slate.com/id/2114925/.

11. Greenberg SD. *Hello Darkness, My Old Friend*. Brentwood, TN: Post Hill Press, 2020, page 117.

4. Scientific Discoveries in Dreams: Sleeping While the Mind Works

1. Heraclitus, quoted in Marcus Aurelius. *Meditations*. Staniforth M, translator. New York: Penguin, 2004, page 69, item 42.

2. Marcus Aurelius. *Meditations*. Staniforth M, translator. New York: Penguin, 2004, page 10.

3. Browne MW. "The benzene ring: dream analysis." *The New York Times*, August 16, 1988. Viewed at https://www.nytimes.com/1988/08/16/science/the-benzene-ring-dream-analysis.html.

4. Jung CG. *The Psychology of Transference*. Princeton: Princeton University Press, 1969, pages 4–5. Viewed at The Internet Archive at https://archive.org/details/psychologyoftran00jung/page/n1/mode/2up.

5. Jung CG. "Approaching the unconscious," in Jung CG, von Franz M-L, Henderson JL, Jacobi J, and Jaffé A. *Man and his Symbols*. Garden City, NY: Doubleday, 1964 (posthumous), page 38.

6. Sacks O. *Uncle Tungsten: Memories of a Chemical Boyhood.* New York: Vintage Books, 2001, pages 198–199.

7. Mazzarello P. "What dreams may come?" *Nature* 2000; 408:523.

8. Agassiz ECC. *Louis Agassiz: His Life and Correspondence.* Cambridge, MA, 1885. Project Gutenberg eBook, 2020 update, eBook # 6078, pages 76–77. Viewed at https://www.gutenberg.org/cache/epub/6078/pg6078.html.

9. Loewi O. "An autobiographical sketch." *Perspectives in Biology and Medicine* 1960; 4:3–25.

10. Kanigel R. *The Man Who Knew Infinity: A Life of the Genius Ramanujan.* New York: Washington Square Press, 1991, pages 36, 98, 281.

11. Rocke AJ. "Kekulé's 'dreams,'" in *Image and Reality: Kekulé, Kopp, and the Scientific Imagination.* Chicago: University of Chicago Press, 2010, pages 293–323.

12. Ghibellini R and Meier B. "The hypnagogic state: A brief update." *J. Sleep Res.* 2023; 32: e13719. Doi: 10.1111jsr.13719.

5. Will DNA be the Next Invisible Ink?

1. Church GM, Gao Y, Kosuri S. "Next-generation digital information storage in DNA." *Science* 2012; 337:1628.

2. Goldman N, Bertone P, Chen S, et al. "Towards practical, high-capacity, low-maintenance information storage in synthesized DNA." *Nature* 2013; 494:77–80.

3. Hysolli E. "A DNA synthesis and decoding strategy tailored for storing and retrieving digital information." Wyss Institute website, Harvard University. August 6, 2019. Viewed at https://wyss.harvard.edu/news/save-it-in-dna/.

4. Ionkov L, Settlemyer B. "DNA: The ultimate data-storage solution." *Scientific American*, May 28, 2021. https://www.scientificamerican.com/article/dna-the-ultimate-data-storage-solution/.

5. Reitsema LJ, Mittnik A, Kyle B, et al. "The diverse genetic origins of a Classical period Greek army." *PNAS* 2022. Viewed at pnas.org/doi/pdf/10.1073/pnas.2205272119.

6. Fan C, Deng Q, Zhu TF. "Bioorthogonal information storage in L-DNA with a high-fidelity mirror-image *Pfu* DNA polymerase." *Nature Biotechnology* 2021; 39:1548–1555.

6. Research Opportunities for Medical Students and Residents

1. Rothberg MB. Overcoming the obstacles to research during residency: What does it take? *JAMA* 2012; 308:2191–2192.

2. Steckelberg JM, Vlietstra RE, Ludwig J, Mann RJ. Werner Forssmann (1904–1979) and his unusual success story. *Mayo Clin Proc* 1979; 54:746–748.

3. Ladewig PP. Nobel laureate Werner Forssmann. *Mayo Clin Proc* 1980; 55:195(lett).

4. Marshall B. Helicobacter pylori & peptic ulcer. In Bynum W and Bynum H, eds. *Great Discoveries in Medicine*. London: Thames and Hudson, 2011, pages 288–291.

5. Rosenthal SM. An improved method for using phenoltetrachlorphthalein as a liver function test. *J Pharmaco & Exper Therap* 1922; 19:385–391.

6. Rosenthal SM and White EC. Clinical application of the bromsulphalein test for hepatic function. *JAMA* 1925; 84:1112–1114.

7. Tabor CW and Tabor H. It all started on a streetcar in Boston. *Ann Rev Biochem* 1999; 68:1–32.

8. Bliss M. *The Discovery of Insulin*. Chicago: University of Chicago Press, 1982.

7. The Origins of NIH Medical Research Grants

1. National Institutes of Health. NIH RePORT [*sic*]: Budget and spending: Research grants. 2022. Table

101. Viewed at https://report.nih.gov/funding/
nih-budget-and-spending-data-past-fiscal-years/
budget-and-spending.

2. National Institutes of Health. What we do: Budget. National Institutes of Health website, 2022. Viewed at https://www.nih.gov/about-nih/what-we-do/budget.

3. Harden VA. *Inventing the NIH: Federal Biomedical Research Policy, 1887–1937*. Baltimore: The Johns Hopkins University Press, 1986.

4. Mandel R. *A Half Century of Peer Review: 1946–1996*. Bethesda: Division of Research Grants, National Institutes of Health, 1996.

5. Schneider WH. The origin of the medical research grant in the United States: The Rockefeller Foundation and the NIH extramural funding program. *J. Hist. Med. Allied Sci.* 2015; 70(2):279–311.

6. Swain DC. The rise of a research empire, 1930 to 1950. *Science* 1962; 138(3546):1233–1237.

7. Willcox AW. The Public Health Service Act, 1944. *Bulletin*, August 1944, pages 15–17. Viewed at Social Security Administration website, https://www.ssa.gov/policy/docs/ssb/v7n8/v7n8p15.pdf.

8. Strickland SP. *The Story of the NIH Grants Programs*. Lanham, MD: University Press of America, 1989.

9. Schmidt CF. Alfred Newton Richards, 1876–1966, a biographical memoir. *Biographical Memoirs*. National Academy of Sciences, National Academy Press, Washington, DC, 1971, pages 271–318.

10. Van Slyke CJ. New horizons in medical research. *Science* 1946; 104(2711): 559–567.

11. Bureau of Labor Statistics. CPI [Consumer Price Index] inflation calculator. Viewed at https://www.bls.gov/data/inflation_calculator.htm.

12. National Institutes of Health. Commonly asked questions about equipment under grants. *NIH Guide for Grants and Contracts*, vol. 24, no. 15, April 28, 1995. Viewed at https://grants.nih.gov/grants/guide/notice-files/not95-121.html.

13. Miles RE, Jr. *The Department of Health, Education, and Welfare*. New York: Praeger, 1974.

14. Center for Scientific Review, NIH. CSR data and evaluations. 2022. Viewed at https://public.csr.nih.gov/AboutCSR/Evaluations.

15. Heniff B, Jr. The Federal Fiscal Year. Report for Congress 98–325. Congressional Research Service, 2008. Viewed at https://budgetcounsel.files.wordpress.com/2016/11/98-325.pdf.

16. National Institutes of Health. NIH Grants & Funding: NIH Research Project Grant Program (R01). 2022. Viewed at https://grants.nih.gov/grants/funding/r01.htm.

17. NIH Center for Scientific Review. Center for Scientific Review website, 2022. Viewed at https://www.csr.nih.gov/RevPanelsAndDates/RevDates.aspx.

18. Endicott KM and Allen EM. The growth of medical research 1941–1953 and the role of Public Health Service research grants. *Science* 1953; 118(3065): 337–343.

8. Medical Misinformation and "The Bellman's Fallacy" in the Internet Era

1. Carroll L. "The Hunting of the Snark," in Gardiner M, ed. *The Annotated Snark*. Harmondsworth, UK: Penguin Books, 1962, page 46. First published 1876.

2. Gardiner M, ed. *The Annotated Snark*. Harmondsworth, UK: Penguin Books, 1962, pages 46–47, footnote 7.

3. Skrabanek P and McCormick J. *Follies and Fallacies in Medicine*. Buffalo: Prometheus Books, 1990, pages 36–37.

4. Waldron HA. "Hippocrates and lead." *Lancet* 1973; 2:626 (letter).

5. Stolley PD and Lasky T. "The Bellman always rings thrice." *Ann. Int. Med.* 1993; 118:158 (letter).

6. Sahni NR and Carrus B. "Artificial intelligence in U.S. health care delivery." *N Engl J Med* 2023; 389:348-358.

7. Densen P. Challenges and opportunities facing medical education. *Trans Am Clin Climatol Assoc* 2011; 122:48–58.

8. Google search performed on August 24, 2023.

9. Kahneman D. *Thinking, Fast and Slow.* New York: Farrar, Straus and Giroux, 2011, page 62.

Shakespeare

9. When Paintings of Shakespeare's Plants Were Found Behind a Shelf of Books

1. Tabor, E. Plant poisons in Shakespeare. *Economic Botany* 1970; 24:1:81–94.

2. Towne, RM. *Plant Lore of Shakespeare.* Louisville, KY: The Frame House Gallery, 1974.

10. A Shakespeare Expert on the Internet, by Surprise

1. Tabor, E. Plant poisons in Shakespeare. *Economic Botany* 1970; 24:1:81–94.

11. Plant Poisons in Shakespeare

1. All Shakespeare quotations are from Harrison GB, ed. *Shakespeare – The Complete Works.* New York: Harcourt, Brace & World, 1952.

2. Gerarde J. *The Herball or Generall Historie of Plantes.* London: Norton, 1597.

3. Bankes R (publisher). *An Herball* (known as "Bankes' *Herbal*"), London: Bankes, 1525. Reprinted: Larkey SV and Pyles T, eds. New York: New York Botanical Garden, 1941.

4. Larkey SV. Introduction. In 1941 reprint of Bankes, 1525, pages X-XI.

5. Rohde ES. *The Old English Herbals*. London: Longmans, Green, 1922, pages 204–206.

6. Turner, W. *Herbal*. Collen (Cologne): Arnold Birckman, 1568 [this was the first edition that combined parts 1, 2, and 3 of this herbal].

7. Langham, W. *The Garden of Health*. London: "Deputies of C. Barker," 1597. [Later editions published by Harper; in some copies, the publication date is misprinted as 1579.]

8. Monardes, D. *Joyfull Newes Out of the New-Found Worlde*. Frampton J, translator. London: Allde, 1596.

9. Brown I. *Shakespeare*. New York: Time, 1962, page 61.

10. Rohde, 1922, page 118.

11. Rohde, 1922, pages 102, 118.

12. Brown, 1962, page 39.

13. Brown, 1962, pages 60–61.

14. Brown, 1962, pages 179–180.

15. For instance, Gerarde, 1597, page 824; Langham, 1597, pages 288, 547; and others.

16. Suggested by Harrison, 1952, page 1191, footnote to line 84.

17. Larkey, 1941, page XX.

18. Gerarde, 1597, Latin index, see "Conion."

A few of the citations for this essay have been updated for this volume using more recent bibliographical findings.

The reprinting of this article is dedicated to Professor Richard Evans Schultes (1915–2001) of Harvard University, whose devotion to botany and teaching inspired this work.

12. The Politician Who Loved Shakespeare

1. Schlesinger AM, Jr. *Robert Kennedy and His Times.* New York: Ballantine Books, 1978, page 882.

2. Tye L. *Bobby Kennedy: The Making of a Liberal Icon.* New York: Random House, 2016, page 377.

3. Schlesinger 1978, pages 665–668.

4. Thomas E, *Robert Kennedy: His Life.* New York: Simon & Schuster, 2000, page 345.

5. Kennedy R.F. Speech to the Democratic National Convention. In: Guthman EO, Allen CR, eds. *RFK: Collected Speeches.* New York: Viking, 1993, pages 115–117.

6. Gwirtzman M. Oral history, 1972. Website of the John F. Kennedy Presidential Library and Museum. Viewed at https://www.jfklibrary.org/sites/default/files/archives/RFKOH/Gwirtzman%2C%20Milton%20S/RFKOH-MSG-03/RFKOH-MSG-03-TR.pdf

7. Townsend KK. Speech at conference titled, "Robert F. Kennedy and the 1968 Campaign," March 16, 2008. Website of the John F. Kennedy Presidential Library and Museum. Viewed at https://www.jfklibrary.org/events-and-awards/forums/past-forums/transcripts/robert-f-kennedy-and-the-1968-campaign.

8. All quotations of Shakespeare's works, unless otherwise referenced, are from: Harrison GB, ed. *Shakespeare: The Complete Works.* New York: Harcourt, Brace & World, 1952.

9. Townsend KK. Remarks in memory of Robert F. Kennedy, Arlington National Cemetery, June 6, 2018. Viewed at http://www.rfkspeeches.com/50[th]_townsend/

10. Thomas 2000, pages 17–18.

11. Whittaker J. Eulogy. In: Salinger P, Guthman E, Mankiewicz F, Seigenthaler J, eds. *An Honorable Profession: A Tribute to Robert F. Kennedy.* New York: Doubleday, 1968, pages 106–107.

12. Tabor E. Personal recollections. The author worked in the Senate office of Robert F. Kennedy in the summers of 1965, 1966, and 1967.

13. Harrison GB. "The Tragedy of Coriolanus: Introduction." In Harrison GB, ed. *Shakespeare: The Complete Works.* New York: Harcourt, Brace & World, 1952, pages 1265–1269.

14. Shakespeare's Bilingual Play

1. All quotations of Shakespeare's works, unless otherwise referenced, are from: Harrison GB, ed. *Shakespeare: The Complete Works.* New York: Harcourt, Brace & World, 1952.

2. There are a total of 23 scenes in *Henry V.*

15. Shakespeare and Memory

1. All quotations of Shakespeare's works, unless otherwise referenced, are from: Harrison GB, ed. *Shakespeare: The Complete Works.* New York: Harcourt, Brace & World, 1952.

2. Word counts are from: George Mason University. *Open Source Shakespeare,* 2021 edition. Viewed at https://opensourceshakespeare.org.

3. Aristotle. *De Anima.* 429 b 22. 480 a 9. Hicks RD, translator. Cambridge, UK: Cambridge University Press, 1907. Viewed at Internet Archive at https://archive.org/stream/aristotledeanima005947mbp/aristotledeanima005947mbp_djvu.txt.

Historical Moments

17. Harvard Scholars in English

1. Bate WJ, Shinagel M, Engell J. *Harvard Scholars in English, 1890 to 1990.* Cambridge, MA: Harvard University Press, 1991.

2. Unger SJ. "Bullitt to resign as Quincy master." *The Harvard Crimson*, September 28, 1965. Viewed at https://www.thecrimson.com/article/1965/9/28/bullitt-to-resign-as-quincy-master/.

3. Vaillant GE. *Triumphs of Experience: The Men of the Harvard Grant Study.* Cambridge, MA: Belknap Press, 2012.

4. Hamid RD and Schisgall EJ. "As Harvard axes shopping week, students opt to create their own." *The Harvard Crimson*, February 3, 2023. Viewed at https://www.thecrimson.com/article/2023/2/3/diy-shopping-week/#:~:text=Following%20years%20of%20fierce%20and,to%20formally%20enroll%20in%20them.

18. The Mystery Plaque

Sources

Baglione JM "Bridge of sorrow, by way of Faulkner." *The Harvard Gazette*, July 20, 2017.

Crinkley R. "William Faulkner: The Southern mind meets Harvard in the era before World War I." [Obituary] *The Harvard Crimson*, July 12, 1962. Viewed at https://www.thecrimson.com/article/1962/7/12/william-faulkner-the-southern-mind-meets/.

Houghteling N. "Expos students embark on literary scavenger hunt." *The Harvard Crimson*, May 6, 2004.

Russakoff D. "Faulkner and the bridge to the South." *The Washington Post*, July 21, 1985.

Siliezar J. "In search of Quentin Compson." *The Harvard Gazette*, June 27, 2019.

19. Long Before Pearl Harbor, an Entire Hospital Was Sent to Help England in World War II

1. Gordon JE. "The Harvard Unit in London." *Harvard Alumni Bulletin*, Oct. 5, 1940, p. 19–21.

2. Jaqua MA. Letters of Mary Alice Jaqua, 1940–1945. The Mary Alice Jaqua Papers, a file in the Ella Strong Denison Library, Special Collections at Claremont Colleges, Claremont, CA.

3. Houser GF. "Harvard and the Red Cross in England." *Harvard Alumni Bulletin*, October 4, 1941, pages 16–18.

4. Jaqua, 1940–1945.

5. Jaqua, 1940–1945.

6. Various documents, including article reprints. From a bound file titled, *Clippings – Harvard-Red Cross Unit – England – 1940–1942.* Countway Library, Harvard University, Boston, MA.

7. Vivette PB. "The United Kingdom." In Lada J and Hoff EC, eds. *Preventive Medicine in World War II, Volume VIII.* Washington, DC: Office of the Surgeon General, United States Army, 1976, pages 375–376.

8. Gordon, 1940.

Acknowledgements: Thanks to the Center for the History of Medicine, Countway Library, Harvard University, Boston, MA; the Ella Strong Denison Library, Scripps College, Claremont, CA; and the Himmelfarb Health Sciences Library, The George Washington University, Washington, DC.

20. A Harvard Class in World War II

1. Bethell JT. *Harvard Observed: An Illustrated History of the University in the Twentieth Century.* Cambridge, MA: Harvard University Press, 1998, pages 133–172.

2. Tabor, E. "Long before Pearl Harbor, an entire hospital was sent to help England in World War II." *Hektoen Int.*, spring 2022. Viewed at: https://hekint.org/2022/05/26/long-before-pearl-harbor-an-entire-hospital-was-sent-to-help-england-in-world-war-ii/.

3. Harvard Class of 1937. *Triennial Report – 1940.* Boston, 1940.

   In that era, the first reunion for each class occurred three years after graduation instead of the five-year interval that was used later.

   In addition to autobiographical essays, this volume contains biographical summaries written by family members or reunion staff for classmates who did not respond to essay requests or who were deceased.

4. Keller M. and Keller P. *Making Harvard Modern: The Rise of America's University.* New York: Oxford University Press, 2001, page 165.

5. Crimson News Staff. "College life during World War II based on country's military needs." *The Harvard Crimson*, December 7, 1956. Viewed at https://www.thecrimson.com/article/1956/12/7/college-life-during-world-war-ii/.

6. Harvard Class of 1937. *Decennial Report of the Harvard Class of 1937.* Cambridge, MA, 1947.

   In addition to autobiographical essays, this volume contains biographical summaries written by family members or reunion staff for classmates who did not respond to essay requests or who were deceased. In addition, some information in this volume was obtained by the reunion staff in 1947 from the "Harvard War Records Office" that existed during World War II.

7. Crimson News Staff. "24,476 Harvard men now in U.S. services." *The Harvard Crimson*, January 23, 1945. Viewed at https://www.thecrimson.com/article/1945/1/23/24476-harvard-men-now-in-us/#:~:text=Figures%20complete%20through%20January%206,Harvard%20Alumni%20Association%20announced%20yesterday.

This article states that as of January 23, 1945, 24,476 alumni had served in the armed forces during World War II, which is possibly the latest published statistic for Harvard alumni serving in World War II.

22. The Obituary Reader

1. Hall D. *Essays After Eighty*. Boston: Houghton Mifflin Harcourt, 2014, page 90.

2. Most of these obituaries appeared in *The Washington Post*.

23. Obituaries of Spies

1. Most of these obituaries appeared in *The Washington Post*.

24. African Slaves in the North

Sources

Brown TH. "The African connection: Cotton Mather and the Boston smallpox epidemic of 1721–1722." *J Am Med Assoc* 1988; 260:2247–2249.

Chestnut M. in Woodward CV, ed. *Mary Chestnut's Civil War*. New Haven: Yale University Press, 1981, page 201.

Comfort WW. *William Penn, 1644–1718: A Tercentenary Estimate.* Philadelphia: University of Pennsylvania Press, 1944, pages 152–153.

Crimaldi L. "Harvard Confronts its History of Slavery," *The Boston Globe*, March 4, 2017. Viewed at https://www.bostonglobe.com/metro/2017/03/03/

harvard-confronts-its-history-slavery-conference/
rhnOAfoCXbWuVniV1vMpcO/story.html .

Desrochers RE, Jr. "Slave-for-sale advertisements and slavery
in Massachusetts, 1704–1781. *The William and Mary
Quarterly* 2002; 59:623–664. Viewed at https://www.jstor.
org/stable/3491467?seq=1#page_scan_tab_contents.

Fenn EA. *Pox Americana: The Great Smallpox Epidemic of
1775–82.* New York: Hill and Wang, 2001.

Goodwin DK. *Team of Rivals: The Political Genius of Abraham
Lincoln.* New York: Simon and Schuster, 2005, pages 30–31.

Greene LJ. *The Negro in Colonial New England, 1620–1776.*
New York: Columbia University Press, 1942. Reprinted by
Martino Fine Books, Eastford, CT, 2017.

Krantz L. "Harvard Unveils Plaque in Memory of Slaves," *The
Boston Globe*, April 6, 2016. Viewed at https://www.
bostonglobe.com/metro/2016/04/06/harvard-unveil-
plaque-memory-slaves/pjc6lmg8HY0awonqLLE2EP/
story.html .

McManus EJ. *Black Bondage in the North.* Syracuse: Syracuse
University Press, 1973.

Moore FD. "Muddy River and Boylston's 250th," *N Engl J Med*
1971; 284:1438–1439. Viewed at http://www.nejm.org/
doi/full/10.1056/NEJM197106242842514.

25. Two Great European Writers Who Were Descendants of African Slaves

DUMAS

Hemmings FWJ. *The King of Romance: A Portrait of
Alexandre Dumas*. London: Hamish Hamilton, 1979.

Lucas-Dubreton J. *The Fourth Musketeer: The Life of
Alexander [sic] Dumas.* New York: Coward-McCann,
1928.

Pushkin

Binyon TJ. *Pushkin: A Biography*. New York: Alfred A.
Knopf, 2003.

Massie RK. *Peter the Great: His Life and World*. New York:
Ballantine Books, 1980.

Nepomnyashchy CT, Svobodny N, and Trigos LA, eds. *Under
the Sky of My Africa: Alexander Pushkin and Blackness*.
Evanston: Northwestern University Press, 2006.

26. Time and Punishment

1. The works of Heraclitus have only survived in the form
of quotations cited by other people in ancient times. This
statement by Heraclitus survived because it was quoted
by Plato in the form shown here immediately before the
superscript. From: Plato. *Cratylus*. Jowett B, translator.
Project Gutenberg. Viewed at https://www.gutenberg.org/
files/1616/1616-h/1616-h.htm.

2. Aurelius M. *Meditations*. Staniforth M, translator. New
York: Penguin Books, page 39.

3. Knox, B. *Backing into the Future: The Classical Tradition
and Its Renewal*. New York: W.W. Norton, 1994, pages
11–12.

4. *The Revelation of Saint John the Divine*. Rev 1:8. King James
Version.

5. Isaacson, W. *Einstein: His Life and Universe*. New York:
Simon & Schuster, 2007, page 540.